NEONATAL
INTENSIVE CARE MANUAL

NEONATAL
INTENSIVE CARE MANUAL

RICHARD P. WENNBERG, M.D.

Professor of Pediatrics
Division of Neonatology
Department of Pediatrics
University of California at Davis
School of Medicine
Davis, California

BOYD W. GOETZMAN, M.D., PH.D.

Associate Professor of Pediatrics
Chief, Division of Neonatology
Department of Pediatrics
University of California at Davis
School of Medicine
Davis, California

YEAR BOOK MEDICAL PUBLISHERS, INC.
CHICAGO

0   9   8   7   6   5   4   3   2   1

Library of Congress Cataloging in Publication Data

Wennberg, Richard P.
    Neonatal intensive care manual.

    Includes bibliographies and index.
    1. Neonatal intensive care—Handbooks, manuals, etc.
2. Infants (Newborn)—Diseases—Treatment—Handbooks,
manuals, etc.   I. Goetzman, Boyd W.   II. Title.   [DNLM:
1. Critical Care—in infancy & childhood—handbooks.
2. Intensive Care Units, Neonatal—handbooks.   3. Neonatology—handbooks.   WS 39 W476n]
RJ253.5.W46   1985   618.92'01   84–17326
ISBN 0–8151—9219–3

Sponsoring editor: Diana L. McAninch
Editing supervisor: Frances M. Perveiler
Production project manager: Sharon W. Pepping
Proofroom supervisor: Shirley E. Taylor

NOTICE

Every effort has been made to ensure that the drug dosage schedules herein are accurate and in accord with the standards accepted at the time of publication. However, as new research and experience broaden our knowledge, changes in treatment and drug therapy occur. Therefore, the reader is advised to check the product information sheet included in the package of each drug he plans to administer to be certain that changes have not been made in the recommended dose or in the contraindications. This is of particular importance in regard to new or infrequently used drugs.

PREFACE

THE "HOUSE OFFICER MANUAL" for the Neonatal Intensive Care Unit had its inception in 1975 when it became apparent that many physicians in training, such as residents in obstetrics, anesthesiology, and family practice, would have but a brief opportunity to learn the fundamentals of newborn stabilization and care. Since then the manual has grown continuously in size and information, resulting in the current edition, the first to be published.

This handbook is *not* a text book; it is intended to be used as a quick reference for procedures and acceptable approaches to problems encountered in our Newborn Intensive Care Unit at the University of California, Davis Medical Center. For the inexperienced, the manual should facilitate orientation to newborn intensive care. For the more senior residents, it should serve as a refresher for common routines, dosages, and normal values as well as an immediate guide for managing new problems. For neither should it be considered the final word nor the totality of reading experience required to gain competence in newborn care.

While guidelines to the clinical management of neonatal disease have become relatively uniform between institutions in recent years, each nursery has its own unique resources and approach to specific problems. The manual is to a large extent a distillation of current recipes and reference values, and will require continued revision as new information emerges. Unfortunately, many of the recommendations are of necessity rather arbitrary and based on "experience" rather than on the results of convincing clinical research. It can only be hoped that the acquisition of new knowledge through continued clinical and basic research will eventually render both the problems and their recommended therapeutic approaches obsolete. In the meantime we hope this will prove to be a practical resource to facilitate patient care and teaching and would welcome suggestions which might improve future editions.

We are deeply indebted to the Manual's contributors who

not only provide the written word but spend many hours in the Newborn Intensive Care Unit assisting in the care of our patients. This dialogue is critical to advancing the science as well as the quality of newborn care. Many have contributed to the Manual by their review and comments. We would particularly like to acknowledge the assistance of our colleagues Jay Milstein, M.D., and Charles Ahlfors, M.D., for their involvement in all phases of this project, and for their constructive criticism; to Mead Johnson Nutritional Division for printing the precursor of this manual during the past three years; to Cece Price and Pat Peacock for typing (and retyping) the manuscript; and to the indispensible Julie Dunn, who spent many hours in organizing, proofreading and editing the manual, and without whom the project may never have been completed.

RICHARD P. WENNBERG, M.D.
BOYD W. GOETZMAN, M.D., PH.D.

Contents

1

Premature Labor and Delivery

A. SOME RISK FACTORS FOR PREMATURITY AND THEIR MANAGEMENT

Nearly 8% of all pregnant women in the United States deliver prematurely. Despite the development of effective medication to suppress uterine activity, the majority of patients in premature labor are not candidates for therapy. Ultimately, effective identification of the pregnancy at risk and institution of prenatal therapy may have a greater impact on perinatal outcome.

1. **Socioeconomic Status** Nutritional counseling and assistance, sociological and educational reform.

2. **Smoking** Mass education, cessation.

3. **Unwanted Pregnancy** Family planning.

4. **Hypertension, Anemia, Diabetes** Preconception diagnosis and treatment.

5. **Urinary Infection** Antibiotic therapy.

6. **Repetitive Abortion** Hysterosalpingogram and treatment as indicated.

7. **Incompetent Cervix** Cerclage at 14 to 16 weeks' gestation.

8. **Multiple Gestation** Prophylactic bed rest, prophylactic tocolysis.

9. **Abdominal Surgery** Preoperative and postoperative monitoring of uterine activity.

10. **Iatrogenic Prematurity** Objective documentation of gestational age by ultrasound, amniotic fluid analysis, or both prior to elective delivery.

1

11. **Unknown Causes** (responsible for majority of cases) Future research.

12. **Premature Rupture of Membranes (PROM)** One of the leading causes.

  a. Diagnosis
    i. History of leaking fluid, "gush" of fluid.
    ii. Diagnostic triad of PROM
      a) Vaginal pool of fluid.
      b) Positive nitrazine test result (amniotic fluid and blood are alkaline; vaginal secretions are acid).
      c) Amniotic fluid produces arborization (ferning) pattern on microscopic smear.
    iii. Additional tests
      a) Amniotic fluid tests (e.g., lecithin:sphingomyelin [LIS] ratio, phosphatidyl glycerol).
      b) Cervical culture, look for group B β streptococcus and gonococcus.

  b. Etiologic factors are poorly understood.

  c. A management algorithm for patients with PROM is depicted in Figure 1–1. The roles of prophylactic antibiotics and steroids in the management of PROM remain controversial, as does the impact of PROM on the incidence of respiratory distress syndrome (RDS).

B. TOCOLYTIC AGENTS

Increased success in caring for infants weighing less than 1,000 gm (<28 weeks) has led to more aggressive maternal-fetal therapy.

1. **Tocolysis Is Most Effective**

  a. Between 28 and 36 weeks' gestation.

  b. No chorioamnionitis, maternal or fetal compromise.

  c. Cervical dilatation is less than 4 cm.

2. **Bed Rest and Hydration**

  a. Increases uterine perfusion with left uterine displacement.

  b. Should be the first step in tocolytic therapy.

3. **Magnesium Sulfate (MGSO$_4$)** is often the agent of first choice.

  a. Interferes with calcium binding in myometrial smooth muscle.

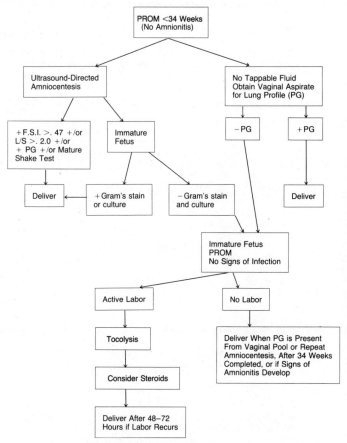

Fig 1–1.—Management algorithm for patients with premature rupture of membranes (PROM). FSI indicates foam stability index; L/S, lecithin/sphingomyelin ratio; PG, phosphatidyl glycerol.

    b. Maternal side effects
       i. Nausea, headache, palpitation.
       ii. Respiratory depression.
       iii. Hypothermia.
    c. Fetal side effects
       i. Hypotonia—common. Often leads to lower Apgar scores.

ii. Respiratory depression—common if maternal magnesium level is greater than 6 mg/dl.

iii. Convulsions—rare.

4. **β-Adrenergic Agents**   stimulate the β receptors of the sympathetic nervous system, producing uterine and bronchial smooth-muscle relaxation as well as peripheral vasodilation and tachycardia.

a. Isoxsuprine—first agent available.

b. Terbutaline—used experimentally in many centers.

c. Ritodrine—the *only* agent currently approved by the FDA for use in inhibiting premature labor. (The following information holds for all β-mimetics.)

   i. Maternal side effects

     a) Tachycardia, palpitations, restlessness

     b) Widened pulse pressure

     c) Transient hypokalemia

     d) Hyperglycemia

     e) Hemodilution

     f) Premature ventricular contractions (PVCs)

     g) Angina-like chest pain

     h) Pulmonary edema

   ii. Fetal side effects

     a) Tachycardia

     b) Hypoglycemia

     c) Hypocalcemia

     d) Blood volume expansion

5. **Other Drugs Previously or Currently Considered**

a. Ethanol—inhibits release of oxytocin from the pituitary.

b. Indomethacin and aspirin derivatives inhibit synthesis of prostaglandins involved in initiation of labor.

c. Progestational agents relax uterine smooth muscle and may be useful for prophylaxis.

C. **MATERNAL STEROID ADMINISTRATION** is used to accelerate fetal lung maturity and to reduce the incidence of neonatal RDS.

1. **Controversial**   We continue to use glucocorticoids before 33 weeks, in selected patients beyond 32 weeks, and with PROM when amniotic fluid analysis indicates immaturity (e.g., ratio < 1.8).

2. **Therapeutic Regimen** Dexamethasone, 12 mg intramuscularly (IM) every 12 hours for two to four doses.

3. *Possible* **Adverse Effects** identified in animal studies are as follows:

   a. Reduced lung growth.

   b. Reduced brain weight secondary to inhibition of cell multiplication.

   c. Decreased immune responsiveness.

4. **Long-Term Human Follow-Up Studies** have failed to expose any neurological, intellectual, or developmental sequelae attributable to steroid (betamethasone, dexamethasone) exposure in utero.

D. INTRAPARTUM MANAGEMENT OF THE PREMATURE INFANT may have a tremendous influence on outcome.

1. **Vaginal Delivery** remains the standard for premature vertex presentations, including vertex/vertex twins.

   a. Continuous electronic monitoring is essential.

   b. Avoid long labors (>12 hours) and head trauma.

2. **Cesarean Section**

   a. *May* improve survival in extreme prematurity (<28 weeks) by decreasing asphyxia and cerebral hemorrhage.

   b. Indicated for premature breech presentation, which is more common than at term.

   c. Probably indicated for vertex/breech twins at less than 34 weeks' gestation.

REFERENCE

1. Johnson J.W.C. (ed.): Obstetric aspects of preterm delivery (symposium). *Clin. Obstet. Gynecol.* 23:15–164, 1980.

2

Assessment of Fetal Well-Being

Technological advances have provided an array of tools with which to assess the well-being of the fetoplacental unit.

A. BIOCHEMICAL TESTING

1. **Hormonal Assays** currently have limited clinical applicability.

   a. Estriol (E_3)
      i. A greater than 35% drop from the mean of the three highest consecutive previous values is significant.
      ii. In diabetic pregnancies, a significant drop may precede fetal demise by only one to two days.
      iii. May be useful in postmaturity and as a check of bioelectronic testing.

   b. Pregnancy-associated plasma protein A (PAPP-A) may be a predictor of patients who will develop preeclampsia, premature labor, or antepartum hemorrhage.

   c. Placental protein 5 (PP5) may be a predictor of patients in whom placental abruption will develop.

2. **Amniotic Fluid Tests** are used to assess fetal lung maturity and the relative risk of neonatal RDS.

   a. Foam stability index (FSI)
      i. Serial dilution of ethanol with constant quantity of amniotic fluid (FSI).
      ii. Adequate surfactant stabilizes a foam ring at the meniscus of 47% by volume ethanol-amniotic fluid mixture.
      iii. False-positive results are rare unless specimens are contaminated (blood, meconium, or vaginal secretions).
      iv. Many false-negative results are seen, including cases of polyhydramnios.
      v. FSI value less than 44 indicates a greater than 50% risk of RDS.

b. L/S ratio is the current standard test
   i. Requires time and skilled technicians.
   ii. Ratio of 2.0/1 is a reliable indicator of maturity.
   iii. Two percent false-positive results, usually in diabetic pregnancies.
       a) With an L/S ratio less than 1.5, about 70% develop RDS.
       b) With an L/S ratio between 1.5 and 2.0, about 40% develop RDS.
   v. Not reliable in specimens contaminated by blood, meconium, or vaginal secretions.

c. Phosphatidyl glycerol (PG)
   i. Aids in stabilizing surfactant membrane.
   ii. Virtually no false-positive findings.
   iii. Not affected by blood, meconium, or vaginal contamination.
   iv. Lack of PG does not correlate well with neonatal RDS.

d. Fetal lung profile
   i. Combination of L/S ratio, percent lecithin, PG, and phosphatidylinositol (PI) improves both the false-positive and false-negative rates.
   ii. Costly and time consuming.

B. ELECTRONIC FETAL HEART RATE MONITORING

1. Basic Patterns

a. Baseline fetal heart rate (120 to 160 beats per minute).

b. Fetal tachycardia (>160 beats per minute) may be due to hypoxia or maternal fever.

c. Fetal bradycardia (<120 beats per minute) is usually benign.

2. Fetal Heart Rate Variability (Fig 2–1)

a. Short-term, beat-to-beat irregularity (2 to 3 beats per minute):
   i. Decreased with fetal sleep cycle (20 to 30 minutes), hypoxia, $MGSO_4$, phenobarbitol, narcotics, phenothiazines, general and local anesthetics.
   ii. Correlates well with fetal pH.

b. Long-term—3 to 5 cycles per minute (amplitude of 5 to 20 beats per minute is normal):
   i. Reflected in "waviness" of fetal heart rate tracing.
   ii. Decreased late in the course of hypoxemia.

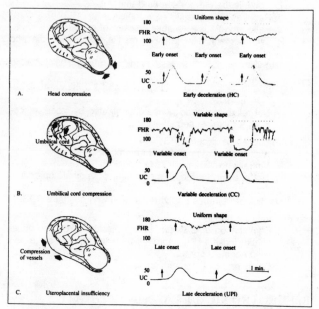

Fig 2–1.—Basic patterns in electronic fetal heart rate (FHR) monitoring. UC indicates uterine contraction; HC, head compression; UPI, uteroplacental insufficiency; CC, cord compression. (From Hon E.H.: An Atlas of Fetal Heart Rate Patterns. New Haven, Conn., Hartley Press, 1968. Used by permission.)

3. Periodic Rate Changes

   a. Accelerations in response to fetal movement:
      i. Usually reassuring.
      ii. Abrupt elevations of 10 to 25 beats per minute above baseline.

   b. Early decelerations secondary to head compression:
      i. Onset near the beginning of the contraction and return to baseline before completion of contraction.
      ii. Least common of periodic changes and uniformly benign.

   c. Variable decelerations caused by umbilical cord compression.
      i. Frequent (approximately 50% of labors).

ii. Abrupt onset and return to baseline during contraction.
iii. May be ominous when severe or associated with tachycardia, loss of beat-to-beat variability, or "overshoot" (a gradual, smooth acceleration lasting more than 30 seconds after a deceleration).

d. Late decelerations:
i. Onset after the apex of the contraction and return to baseline after it is over.
ii. Ominous until proven otherwise.
iii. Correlates well with uteroplacental insufficiency.

C. FETAL MONITORING TECHNIQUES

1. External Instrumentation

a. Doppler Ultrasound
i. The most commonly used method.
ii. Can only interpret long-term variability or an overall decrease in variability.

b. Abdominal fetal ECG
i. When a good signal is obtained, short-term variability is interpretable.

c. Uterine tocodynamometer
i. Records only the interval and duration of contractions, not the strength.

2. Internal instrumentation requires rupture of the membranes.

a. Fetal ECG via scalp electrode
i. Reliable way to analyze both long-term and short-term (beat-to-beat) variability.

b. Uterine-pressure—measuring catheter
i. Quantitates strength of contraction and baseline uterine tone.

D. ANTEPARTUM FETAL TESTING aids in the detection of the fetus in distress and a means of reassuring us that the fetus is doing well.

1. Non–Stress Testing (NST) is based on the observation that fetal heart rate accelerations in association with fetal movement correlate with fetal well-being.

a. Reactive NST—the presence of two accelerations of fetal heart rate, in association with fetal movement of greater than 15 seconds' duration and more than 15 beats per minute above baseline in a 20-minute span.

b. Nonreactive NST—the absence of two accelerations as in a 20-minute span. Follow immediately with contraction stress test to rule out fetal distress.

2. **Contraction Stress Test (CST) or Oxytocin Challenge Test (OCT)** uses the concept of induced contractions to determine the compromised fetus via the presence of late decelerations during fetal monitoring.

a. Contractions can be spontaneous or induced by oxytocin or breast (nipple) stimulation.

b. Negative CST—the absence of late decelerations.

c. Positive CST—consistent and persistent late decelerations with the majority of contractions.

d. Equivocal CST—suspicious uterine hyperstimulation or unsatisfactory contractions.

e. CSTs are now graded as to reactivity as well (reactive if at least one acceleration of 15 beats per minute lasting 15 seconds occurs):
   i. Reactive negative CST—*very* reassuring.
   ii. Nonreactive negative CST—unusual, consider fetal cardiac or CNS abnormality, or drug therapy (phenobarbital, propranolol).
   iii. Reactive positive CST—generally associated with good outcome. Monitor frequently or deliver.
   iv. Nonreactive positive CST—ominous, *rarely* false positive, if greater than 30 weeks' gestation deliver *regardless* of maturity. If less than 30 weeks *may* temporize with biophysical profile testing; individualize management.

E. FETAL ULTRASOUND

1. Gestational Age Assessment

a. Fetal crown-rump length (predictive with ±5 days).

b. Biparietal diameter (BPD) (predictive within ±11 days).

c. Growth-adjusted sonographic age (GASA) using paired BPDs (dating to within ±3–5 days).

d. Fetal femur length (predicts gestational age ±1 week before 24 weeks).

2. **Amniotic Fluid Volume**   Oligohydramnios—fluid absent in most areas of amniotic cavity. May be a good prediction of intrauterine growth retardation or renal agenesis.

3. **Assessment of Fetal Anomalies**   e.g., hydrocephalus, renal or gastrointestinal (GI) tract defects.

F. **BIOPHYSICAL PROFILE**   The value of a profile of tests (fetal breathing, fetal trunk movements, fetal tone or posture, and amniotic fluid volume) in the assessment of fetal well-being is under investigation.

1. When findings from all five tests were normal, perinatal mortality was zero in a recent study.

REFERENCES

1. Cruikshank D.P.: Antepartum fetal surveillance. *Clin. Obstet. Gynecol.* 25:633–804, 1982.
2. Freeman R.J., Garite T.J.: *Fetal Heart Rate Monitoring.* Baltimore, Williams & Wilkins Co., 1981.

3

Resuscitation of the Newborn

Cardiorespiratory depression (heart rate less than 100 beats per minute, hypotension, hypoventilation, or apnea) may occur in 10% to 15% of newborn infants. Prompt therapy may be lifesaving and is necessary to minimize permanent CNS disability.

A. ETIOLOGY OF CARDIORESPIRATORY DEPRESSION

1. **Drugs** With few exceptions, anesthetic and analgesic drugs used in obstetrics cross the placenta and may affect the fetus.

2. **Trauma** Rapid labor, mid-forceps or high-forceps extraction, and breech delivery may be responsible for intracranial hemorrhage or injury. Trauma has decreased in recent years, partly because of the more frequent use of cesarean section for breech presentations and cephalopelvic disproportion.

3. **Hemorrhagic Shock** Fetal blood loss into the mother, into a twin, or from umbilical vessel rupture may be severe. Diagnosis of perinatal blood loss is frequently made only retrospectively after noting a drop in the hematocrit reading.

4. **Intrinsic Cardiac, Pulmonary, or CNS Disease** Anomalies or fetal infection of these key organs can be responsible for cardiorespiratory depression at birth.

5. **Asphyxia** The major cause of cardiorespiratory depression is asphyxia (decreased Po_2 and pH and increased Pco_2).

B. ASPHYXIA

1. Conditions Associated With Asphyxia

   a. A wide range of maternal, fetal, and placental conditions can lead to asphyxia in the newborn.

b. A common factor seems to be marginal exchange of O_2 and CO_2 across the placenta, which becomes further compromised during labor. Oxytocin challenge tests as well as intrapartum fetal monitoring may detect some of those infants who cannot tolerate labor.

2. **Physiology**   Acute total asphyxia (8 to 15 minutes) of animals, followed by resuscitation, has not reproduced the acute clinical symptomatology or long-term CNS sequelae seen in human infants surviving perinatal asphyxia. Experiments in nonhuman primates indicate that more prolonged partial asphyxia (1 to 3 hours) is necessary to reproduce accurately the clinical and pathologic condition most often seen in asphyxiated human infants. Acute asphyxia can produce injury to the basal ganglia and brain stem in primates, but leaves the cerebral cortex intact, a situation rarely encountered in asphyxiated human newborns.

C. RESUSCITATION EQUIPMENT REQUIRED IN THE DELIVERY ROOM   Check presence and function prior to delivery.

1. Overhead radiant warmer

2. Suction source (wall and bulb)

3. Suction catheters

4. Oxygen source

5. Infant resuscitation bag

6. Face masks (assorted sizes)

7. Laryngoscope (with 0 and 1 straight blades)

8. Endotracheal tubes (2.5, 3.0, and 3.5 mm)

9. Umbilical catheterization tray

10. Umbilical catheters (3.5 and 5.0 French)

11. Drugs

12. Syringes, needles, and three-way stopcock

D. RESUSCITATION TECHNIQUE

1. **Thermal Protection** Rapidly wipe the infant dry and place under a radiant heat source.

2. **Position for Airway Management** Place the infant in a left-lateral, head-down tilt position. The supine position promotes airway obstruction.

3. **Pharyngeal Suctioning** Gently suction secretions from the pharynx with a bulb syringe or under direct vision (laryngoscope) with a whistle-tip catheter attached to wall suction or attached to a DeLee Trap using mouth suction. Avoid passing catheters through the nose and into the stomach for the first five minutes of life, as these maneuvers may induce bradycardia.

4. **Airway Suctioning** Thick secretions or meconium may require tracheal suction under direct vision (laryngoscope). On occasion, mouth-to-endotracheal tube suction will be necessary to remove thick meconium from the trachea.

5. **Positive-Pressure Ventilation** Infants with heart rates less than 100 beats per minute need high-quality ventilation with oxygen-enriched gas immediately, as do infants who remain apneic for one minute after birth. With effective ventilation, the heart rate should increase to over 100 beats per minute within 15 to 30 seconds. The first few insufflations may require pressure of 30 to 50 cm of water. Thereafter, lower pressures should suffice unless lung disease is present.

   a. *Bag and mask ventilation*
      i. With the infant's head slightly extended, the mask is grasped with the thumb and first two fingers of the left hand and placed gently but firmly over the infant's mouth and nose. The other two fingers of the left hand are used to support the chin.
      ii. We usually use our continuous positive airway pressure (CPAP) device to deliver oxygen-enriched gas and ventilate newborns.
      iii. A ventilatory rate of 30 to 50 per minute is usually adequate.
      iv. The effectiveness of ventilation is assessed by observation of chest motion and a prompt increase in heart rate. Auscultation of the chest should reveal air entry bilaterally.

v. Gastric distention should be watched for and may be relieved by passing a nasogastric or orogastric tube.

b. *Endotracheal intubation.*—The need for intubation during resuscitation of newborn infants has often been an artifact of the supine position. In this position, the large occiput and tongue and small posterior pharynx combine to produce airway obstruction. Endotracheal intubation is indicated as follows:

i. If bag and mask ventilation is ineffective.
ii. If airway obstruction is suspected (e.g., goiter or micrognathia).
iii. If meconium aspiration is suspected.
iv. If resuscitation is required in patients with abdominal wall defects or diaphragmatic hernia.
v. If external cardiac massage is necessary.

c. The majority of infants with cardiorespiratory depression may be resuscitated by high-quality ventilation alone.

6. **External Cardiac Massage** If the heart rate does not rise above 100 beats per minute within 30 seconds of beginning ventilation, external cardiac massage should be started. Compression, with two fingers, should be over the middle one third of the sternum (Fig 3–1). Lower positions are less effective and may lacerate the liver. A frequency of 100 to 120

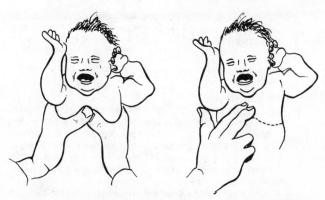

Fig 3–1.—External cardiac massage being performed on a newborn infant. (From Goetzman B.W.: Resuscitation of the newborn, in Niswander K.R. (ed.): Manual of Obstetrics. Boston, Little, Brown & Co., 1980, pp. 389–397. Used by permission.)

compressions per minute is adequate. Depress the sternum 1.5 to 2.0 cm with each compression. Coordination with ventilation seems to be unnecessary. Assess effectiveness by palpating the femoral pulse.

7. Pharmacologic Therapy

a. Catheterization of the umbilical vein with a No. 5 French catheter usually provides the quickest route for administering drugs. Flush drugs through the umbilical catheter with 2 to 3 ml of isotonic saline.

b. If the infant remains pale and bradycardiac for three to five minutes after beginning ventilation, he or she probably has metabolic acidosis and will benefit from the administration of sodium bicarbonate so long as ventilation is adequate. Use a 0.5-mEq/ml concentration and infuse 2 mEq/kg at a rate of 1 to 2 mEq/kg/min or less.

c. If the heart rate does not respond promptly administer epinephrine 1:10,000 (0.1 ml/kg).

d. If the baby still remains bradycardiac administer atropine, 0.01 mg/kg.

e. If hypovolemia is suspected, administer type O rh negative blood cross-matched against the mother, plasmanate or heparinized placental blood (10 to 20 ml/kg), or albumin (1 gm/kg).

f. Subsequent doses of sodium bicarbonate should be based on blood gas analysis. In general, metabolic acidosis with a base deficit of 10 mEq/L or greater should be corrected if the infant's condition remains unstable after resuscitation.

g. Administer other drugs such as 10% calcium gluconate (0.5 ml/kg).

h. Drug depression
   i. Narcotic antagonist, such as naloxone, 0.01 mg/kg, should be administered for suspected drug depression only after appropriate initial resuscitation has taken place and the infant continues to hypoventilate. Too often, a narcotic antagonist is administered in lieu of assisting ventilation, and a wait-and-see attitude prevails to the detriment of the patient.
   ii. Knowledge of maternal heroin use is essential to avoid precipitation of acute narcotic withdrawal.
   iii. Maternal general anesthesia may result in an anesthetized newborn who requires 10 to 15 minutes (occasionally longer) of manual ventilation to recover from the anesthetic.

E. APGAR SCORE

The Apgar score provides a standard for describing the condition of infants at birth. At one and five minutes after birth, five objective signs are evaluated and each is given a score of 0, 1, or 2 (Table 3–1). The sum of the five scores is the Apgar score. A score of 7 to 10 indicates an infant in excellent condition. A score of 3 to 6 indicates moderate depression, and a score of 0 to 2 indicates severe depression. The one-minute Apgar score correlates best with survival, while the five-minute Apgar score seems to be a better prognosticator of neurological damage at 1 year of age.

F. POSTNATAL MANAGEMENT OF ASPHYXIATED INFANTS   Problems to be anticipated include the following:

1. Metabolic Sequelae

a. Lactic acidosis (blood pH less than 7.3 and lactate greater than 2.0 mEq/L) may persist, indicating low cardiac output, poor peripheral perfusion, inadequate oxygenation, or hepatic insufficiency. Alkali therapy or cardiotonic agents such as dopamine may be indicated.

b. Hypoglycemia (blood glucose level lower than 40 mg/dl in full-term infants or less than 30 mg/dl in premature infants) is not uncommon and responds well to glucose infusion at rates of 8 mg/kg/min.

c. Hypocalcemia (serum calcium level less than 8.0 mg/dl in

TABLE 3–1.—APGAR SCORING SYSTEM

SIGN	0	1	2
Heart rate	Absent	<100 bpm*	100+ bpm
Respiratory effort	Absent	Slow, irregular	Good crying
Muscle tone	Flaccid	Flexion of extremities	Active motion; well-flexed extremities
Reflex irritability	No response	Grimace	Vigorous cry
Color	Blue; pale	Body pink; extremities blue	Completely pink

*bpm indicates beats per minute.

term infants or less than 7.0 mg/dl in premature infants) frequently occurs during the second 24 hours of life in asphyxiated infants. The etiology and indications for therapy of hypocalcemia are not well defined. Convulsions or heart failure caused by hypocalcemia should respond to infusion to 200 mg/kg of calcium gluconate over 10 minutes followed by 400 to 500 mg/kg/day.

2. CNS Sequelae

a. Cerebral edema may lead to coma or convulsions. The syndrome of inappropriate antidiuretic hormone secretion may also occur. Assessments of fontanelle tension, cerebral suture width, and head circumference are helpful diagnostically. Fluid infusion in asphyxiated infants should be conservative initially, on the order of 50 ml/kg/day.

b. The use of glucocorticoids, depressive levels of phenobarbital, and osmotic agents is controversial and should be discussed with the attending neonatologist.

c. Cerebral hemorrhage may occur with catastrophic results. If suspected, computed axial tomography or two-dimensional ultrasound studies of the brain are indicated.

3. Renal Sequelae
Acute renal failure is commonly caused by acute tubular necrosis (ATN), less frequently by medullary necrosis, renal cortical necrosis, or renal vein thrombosis. Careful fluid and electrolyte management is required. In ATN, renal function usually improves in three to five days. Occasionally, peritoneal dialysis is necessary.

4. Urinary Bladder
Bladder paralysis is common. It may be necessary to express urine manually from the bladder. Do not confuse this with posterior urethral valves in the male infant.

5. Cardiac Sequelae
Asphyxial cardiac damage may be lethal. Myocardial damage may produce hypotension, low cardiac output, and persistent metabolic acidosis. Roentgenographically, the heart is enlarged, and echocardiography reveals left ventricular dysfunction. Careful fluid management is required, and administration of oxygen, alkali, and occasionally dopamine may be necessary.

6. Pulmonary Sequelae
A variety of pulmonary problems may be precipitated by asphyxia, including pulmonary hypertension, RDS, and impaired lung fluid clearance. When seen together, the term *asphyxial* or *"shock lung"* is often applied.

Sepsis and congenital pneumonia may both contribute to and complicate perinatal asphyxia.

G. OUTCOME   The mortality of severely asphyxiated infants (Apgar 0 to 2) is approximately 50%. Survivors have an increased risk of CNS damage, but it must be remembered that more than 90% will develop normally. Thus, in the absence of serious congenital anomalies, it is prudent to begin resuscitation efforts in severely asphyxiated infants. If an infant does not respond with a sustained increase in heart rate in 15 to 20 minutes, resuscitative efforts may be stopped.

4

Health Care Maintenance

Compulsive attention to caretaking functions of sick and immature infants is critical in assuring optimal outcome. Health care maintenance (HCM) should be attended to daily on work rounds and documented in your problem-oriented progress notes. Maintenance functions must be both monitored and interpreted.

A. CRITICALLY ILL PATIENTS

1. Review and interpret changes in vital signs, including blood pressure (BP).

2. Evaluate temperature fluctuation and neutral thermal environment requirements.

3. Measure and interpret acute weight change (growth vs. fluid balance).

4. Plot weight on Dancis curve and interpret long-term growth pattern (growth vs. fluid balance).

5. Calculate fluid, sodium, potassium, and calcium intakes per kilogram per day.

6. Measure and evaluate serum electrolyte and blood urea nitrogen (BUN) levels. Measure phosphorus and chloride levels at least weekly.

7. Calculate urine output (total and ml/kg/hr). Normal urine output should be 3 to 5 ml/kg/hr.

8. If needed, calculate fluid electrolyte balance using items 3 through 7.

9. Evaluate nutrition. Calculate caloric intake (kcal/kg/day), protein intake (gm/kg/day), and glucose tolerance (mg/kg/min).

10. Review hematocrit reading, urinalysis results, and acid-base status daily.

11. Monitor bilirubin concentration daily until decreasing, and weekly until normal (less than 4 mg/dl).

12. Measure head circumference every other day and plot.

13. Review medications and drug levels where appropriate.

14. Evaluate changes in general activity and behavior.

15. Review problem list.

B. CONVALESCING PATIENTS

1. Review and interpret changes in vital signs.

2. Review appropriateness of thermal environment.

3. Plot weight on Dancis curve and evaluate acute weight change and overall growth pattern.

4. Calculate intake of nutrients (calories/kg, protein/kg).

5. Measure hematocrit reading, BP, urinalysis results, and head circumference weekly.

6. If growth is suboptimal, evaluate electrolyte balance and acid-base status at least weekly.

7. Evaluate changes in clinical status and behavior.

8. Review problem list.

9. Anticipate discharge.

5

Assessment of Gestational Age

A. CLASSIFICATION OF NEWBORNS All newborn admissions should be classified according to maturity and intrauterine growth.

1. **Maturity** Determine gestational age using a modified Dubowitz examination (physical/neurological assessment).

   a. Premature—gestational age less than 37 weeks.

   b. Term—gestational age 37 to 42 weeks.

   c. Postmature—gestational age more than 42 weeks.

2. **Intrauterine Growth** Plot the weight, length, and head circumference vs. the estimated gestational age on the intrauterine growth curve.

   a. Large for gestational age (LGA)—weight above the 90th percentile.

   b. Appropriate for gestational age (AGA)—weight between the 10th and 90th percentiles.

   c. Small for gestational age (SGA)—weight below the 10th percentile.

B. METHOD OF ASSESSMENT: MODIFIED DUBOWITZ EXAMINATION

1. Using a combination of neuromuscular and external physical criteria, gestational age can be estimated independent of obstetric history (Fig 5–1).

2. Accuracy is within two weeks for infants over 30 weeks' gestation. Assessment of gestational age in babies under 30 weeks' gestation is imprecise. Babies are frequently assigned too high a gestational age.

Neuromuscular Maturity

	0	1	2	3	4	5
Posture						
Square Window (wrist)	90°	60°	45°	30°	0°	
Arm Recoil	180°		100°-180°	90°-100°	<90°	
Popliteal Angle	180°	160°	130°	110°	90°	<90°
Scarf Sign						
Heel to Ear						

Physical Maturity

Skin	gelatinous red, trans-parent	smooth pink, vis-ible veins	superficial peeling, &/or rash fuw veins	cracking pale area rare veins	parchment deep cracking no vessels	leathery cracked wrinkled
Lanugo	none	abundant	thinning	bald areas	mostly bald	
Plantar Creases	no crease	faint red marks	anterior transverse crease only	creases ant. 2/3	creases cover entire sole	
Breast	barely percept.	flat areola no bud	stippled areola 1-2mm bud	raised areola 3-4mm bud	full areola 5-10mm bud	
Ear	pinna flat, stays folded	sl. curved pinna; soft c̄ slow recoil	well-curv. pinna; soft but ready recoil	formed & firm c̄ instant recoil	thick cartilage ear stiff	
Genitals ♂	scrotum empty no rugae			testes descend-ing, few rugae	testes down good rugae	testes pendulous deep rugae
Genitals ♀	prominent clitoris & labia minora			majora & minora equally prominent	majora large minora small	clitoris & minora completely covered

MATURITY RATING

Score	Wks.
5	26
10	28
15	30
20	32
25	34
30	36
35	38
40	40
45	42
50	44

Fig 5–1.—Scoring system for simplified clinical assessment of maturation in newborn infants. (From Ballard in [1]. Used by permission.)

3. Notes on Neuromuscular Examination

a. *Posture.*—Assess when the newborn is quiet and supine. Breech babies may have abnormal posturing of lower extremities.

b. *Square window.*—Flex the hand between the thumb and index finger. Do not rotate the wrist. Measure the angle between the hypothenar eminence and forearm.

c. *Arm recoil.*—Hold the forearms flexed for 5 seconds, extend the forearms slowly and release.

d. *Popliteal* angle.—Place the thigh in the knee-chest position with the pelvis flat on the mattress. Extend the lower leg from the knee until resistance is met and measure the angle.

e. *Scarf sign.*—Grasp one hand and try to place it behind the contralateral shoulder, lifting the elbows across the body. See how far the elbow will go across the chest.

f. *Heel to ear.*—With the baby supine, grasp the foot between thumb and index finger and attempt to touch the ipsilateral ear. Note the foot-ear distance and knee extension when resistance is met.

4. **Scoring** Add the total score from the chart and refer to the corresponding score on the maturity rating table in Figure 5–1.

C. LARGE FOR GESTATIONAL AGE INFANTS (LGA)

1. Most LGA infants are simply genetically or nutritionally well endowed, but must be distinguished from infants of diabetic mothers or other conditions with hormonally induced excessive intrauterine growth (e.g., Beckwith's syndrome).

2. Infants of Diabetic Mothers (IDMs)

a. Problems related to carbohydrate homeostasis include the following:

i. Hypoglycemia occurs in most IDMs with nadir at 1 to 2 hours.

ii. In IDMs with marked obesity or a mother with poor control, start intravenous (IV) administration with 10% dextrose in water on admission to avoid panic when the reagent strip (Dextrostix®) indicates hypoglycemia at 1 to 2 hours of age, which is very common.

iii. These patients have problems in glucose mobilization rather than hyperinsulinism at birth, but have β-cell hyperplasia and will overreact to a glucose bolus. Therefore, infuse glucose slowly, and wean from IVs when oral feedings are tolerated.

iv. In general, the more the baby looks like an IDM, the more likely he or she is to have hypoglycemia and the more frequently the baby needs to be monitored with Dextrostix.

b. Hyperbilirubinemia is common. Both the problems of jaundice and hypoglycemia may be ameliorated or prevented by the early introduction of oral nutrition.

c. Hypocalcemia is common in IDMs and may cause jitteriness.

d. IDMs have an increased incidence of several problems:
   i. Congenital anomalies.
   ii. Birth trauma (Erb's palsy, fractured clavicles, head).
   iii. Respiratory disease, particularly transient tachypnea of the newborn and hyaline membrane disease.

D. SMALL FOR GESTATIONAL AGE INFANTS (SGA)

1. Problems Associated with Intrauterine Growth Retardation

a. Maternal hypertension.

b. Maternal uterine abnormalities.

c. Maternal heavy smoking and serious malnutrition are probably additive insults (usually will not cause significant runting alone).

d. Increased likelihood of chromosomal abnormality.

e. Increased incidence of multiple congenital defects of recognizable malformation.

f. Increased likelihood of serious inherited metabolic disease.

g. Increased likelihood of CNS abnormality, developmental delay.

h. Increased likelihood of intrauterine TORCH infection.

2. Diagnostic Evaluation

a. Conduct a physical examination to evaluate problems listed previously.

b. If intrauterine infection is suspected, obtain the following:
   i. Cord blood for IgM level and TORCH titers.
   ii. X-ray films of long bones and posterior-anterior and lateral views of skull.
   iii. Arrange for ophthalmologic evaluation.

c. Evaluate acid-base status and lactate level.

d. Monitor serum glucose level (do not fast infant).

REFERENCES

1. Ballard J.L., Novak K.K., Driver M.: A simplified score for assessment of fetal maturation of newly born infants. J. Pediatr. 95:769–774, 1979.
2. Dubowitz L.M.S., Dubowitz V., Goldberg C.: Clinical assessment of gestational age in the newborn infant. J. Pediatr. 77:1–10, 1970.

6

Temperature Regulation

A. SOURCES OF THERMAL STRESS

1. In the delivery room, wet infants may undergo rapid heat loss due to EVAPORATION.

2. Infants placed on a cold surface may lose heat by CONDUCTION.

3. Infants lose heat by RADIATION when exposed to (but not in contact with) surfaces such as incubator walls or windows with a negative temperature gradient across them.

4. Infants exposed to low ambient temperatures and drafts lose heat by CONVECTION.

5. Hyperthermia may occur if infants are overwarmed, resulting in dire metabolic consequences.

B. NEUTRAL THERMAL ENVIRONMENT

1. *Definition:* Environment (temperature, humidity) at which infants' oxygen consumption is minimal (Figure 6–1).

2. Neutral thermal environmental temperature decreases with increasing gestational age, and postnatal age.

C. MONITORING TEMPERATURE

1. Axillary or abdominal skin temperatures correlate well with oxygen consumption (as opposed to rectal temperatures).

2. The rectal-skin temperature gradient may be useful in distinguishing cold stress from shocklike states.

3. A skin temperature of 36 to 36.5° C is generally satisfactory.

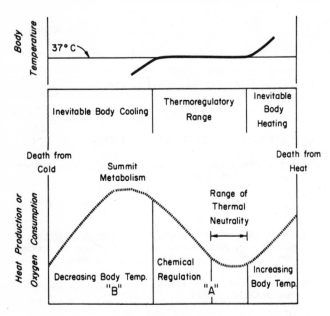

Environmental Temperature

Fig 6–1.—Body temperature of newborn with respect to environmental temperature. (From Klaus M.H., Lanaroff A.A.: Care of the High Risk Neonate. Philadelphia, W.B. Saunders Co., 1973. Used by permission.)

4. Infants with temperature instability may appear stable if on servoregulation. Always evaluate the baby's temperature with respect to environmental temperature (Table 6–1).

D. TEMPERATURE MODULATION

1. **Infants Regulate Temperature by the Following Means:**

   a. Vasodilation and constriction.

   b. Increased metabolism (including brown fat).

   c. Activity.

   d. Adult mechanisms of shivering and sweating are limited or absent in newborns, particularly in premature births.

TABLE 6-1.—Approximate Neutral Thermal Environment
Temperatures*

	weight (GMS) (TEMPERATURE RANGE° C)			
Age	<1200 ±0.5° C	1201–1500 ±0.5° C	1501–2500 ±1.0° C	>2500 (>36 wk) ±1.5° C
0–12 Hr	35.0	34.0	33.3	32.8
12–24 Hr	34.5	33.8	32.8	32.4
24–96 Hr	34.5	33.5	32.3	32.0
4–14 Days		33.5	32.1	32.0
2–3 Wk		33.1	31.7	30.0
3–4 Wk		32.6	31.4	
4–5 Wk		32.0	30.9	
5–6 Wk		31.4	30.4	

*From Scopes, Ahmed: *Arch. Dis. Child* 41:417, 1966. Used by permission.

2. Environment

   a. Infant should be placed in a crib, isolette, or under a radiant
      warmer as appropriate for the infant's size, gestational age,
      illness, and medical care requirements.

   b. Infants in cribs should be swaddled.

   c. Inner shields to reduce radiant heat loss should be consid-
      ered in infants weighing less than 1,000 gm.

   d. Infants should not be removed from isolettes for extended
      periods of time (e.g., procedures, feedings), without provid-
      ing for heat conservation.

E. WITHDRAWAL OF TEMPERATURE
   SUPPORT

   1. Infants are usually larger than 1,500 gm before they can
      maintain their temperatures in an open crib. This is variable.

   2. Attempts to wean an infant who requires an incubator tem-
      perature greater than 30° C usually are unsuccessful.

7

Fluid and Electrolyte Balance

A. GENERAL CONSIDERATIONS

1. Fluid requirements of term vs. permature infants are different due to the variations of the amount and distribution of the total body water with gestational age (Table 7–1).

TABLE 7–1.—DISTRIBUTION OF TOTAL BODY WATER AS PERCENT OF BODY WEIGHT*

WEEKS GESTATION	TOTAL BODY WATER, %	ECW, %	ICW, %
24	86	60	26
28	84	57	27
30	83	55	28
32	82	53	29
34	81	51	30
36	80	49	31
Term	78	45	33

*ECW indicates extracellular water; ICW, intracellular water. (Adapted from Friis-Hansen B. *Amer. J. Clin. Nutr.* 25:1153, 1972.)

2. All newborn infants have abundant extracellular extravascular water. They are expected to excrete the excess and thus lose weight over the first five to seven days of life. The approximate weight loss, as a percent of body weight (BW) is related to gestational age:

GESTATION (WK)	WEIGHT LOSS AS % OF BODY WEIGHT
26	15–20
30	10–15
34	8–10
Term	5–10

3. Premature infants (particularly those below 1,000 gm birth weight) and to a lesser extent term infants, may have excessive water losses over the first days of life due to the following:

   a. High insensible water losses through the skin seen especially in very small infants placed under radiant warmers with low environmental relative humidity.

   b. Phototherapy lights for hyperbilirubinemia may increase insensible water losses from 40 to 50 ml/kg/24 hr to as high as 150 ml/kg/24 hr.

4. Excessive rates of fluid administration have been associated with the following:

   a. Congestive heart failure.

   b. Hyperglycemia (due to glucose load).

   c. Diuresis and electrolyte loss.

5. All of these factors must be considered in calculating fluid requirements and therapy and *must be closely monitored.*

B. GUIDELINES FOR INITIAL FLUID ADMINISTRATION

1. For the first three days of life, the rates (ml/kg/24 hr) of fluid administration shown in Table 7–2 are suggested based on past experience using radiant warmers.

2. High insensible water losses in very small infants under radiant warmers may necessitate IV fluid rates greater than 200 ml/kg/24 hr. It may be desirable to limit insensible water losses using plastic heat shields.

3. If the infant is also taking oral fluid, this volume should be

TABLE 7–2.—BIRTH WEIGHT (GM) GUIDELINES FOR FLUID ADMINISTRATION (ML/KG)

| AGE | BIRTH WEIGHT | | |
	<1,000 gm	1,000–1,500 gm	1,500–2,500 gm
1st 24 hr	100–120	80–100	60–80
2nd 24 hr	120–150	110–130	90–110
> 48 hr	140–180	140–180	120–140

included in the daily input. Distribution between oral and parenteral fluids should maximize caloric intake.

C. ELECTROLYTE REQUIREMENTS

TABLE 7–3.—Electrolyte
Requirements (mEq/kg/24 hr)

	INTRAVENEOUS	ORAL
Sodium	3–5	8
Potassium	3–5	7
Calcium	2	2–3

Routine calcium supplementation is not indicated during the first few days of life unless there is hypocalcemia (a calcium level of less than 6.5 mg/dl in infants weighing less than 1,500 gm or 7.0 mg/dl in infants over 1,500 gm with normal albumin, ECG evidence of hypocalcemia documented by corrected QT interval, or both). The recommended calcium dose for symptomatic hypocalcemia is 200 mg/kg by slow IV push with ECG monitoring (2 mEq of calcium equals 80 mg).

D. MONITORING IV FLUID THERAPY AND ONGOING ADJUSTMENTS

The following assessments of hydration should be obtained as frequently as needed (often every four to six hours in tiny infants with high insensible water loss):

1. Body Weight

2. Blood Chemistries

a. *Sodium.*—(Tends to be lower in premature infants; 130 mEq is acceptable).

b. *Plasma osmolality.*—In the first week of life it must be measured directly. After a week of age, it can be estimated by the following formula.
   $Osm/kg\ water = 5 + 1.86\ Na + 2.8\ BUN + glucose/18$
   (Na in meq/L, BUN and glucose in mg/dl)

c. Serum creatinine and BUN levels reflect renal function and may be elevated over the first 24 hours due to a normally low glomerular filtration rate (GFR) in newborns.

3. Urine

a. *Osmolality.*—(May not be useful in fluid management in the presence of renal, adrenal, or posterior pituitary dysfunction.)

b. *Specific gravity.*—(Proportional to osmolality if no protein or glucose in urine). The osmolality can be estimated from the specific gravity (sp gr) by multiplying the decimal number of the latter by 20:

$$\text{If sp gr} = 1.003, mOsm = 20 \times 3 = 60$$
$$\text{If sp gr} = 1.015, mOsm = 20 \times 15 = 300$$

Reasonable specific gravities are 1.003 to 1.015.

c. The urine sodium level does not assess hydration, but is useful in assessing requirements and, with the serum sodium level, may help to assess fluid and electrolyte needs.

d. Urine volume is typically 50 to 100 cc/kg/24 hr with an osmolality of 75 to 300 mOsm/kg/24 hr if the renal solute load is between 7.5 and 15 mOsm/kg/24 hr.

E. STANDARD RANGES (per kilogram per 24 hours)

1. Water required: 150 ml.

2. Insensible water losses: 40 to 50 ml.

3. Urine output: 48 to 96 ml.

F. INTERPRETATION OF MONITORING INFORMATION

1. An appropriate monitoring period should be decided upon depending on the patient's gestational age and condition (e.g., 4 hours, 12 hours, 24 hours, etc.).

2. Laboratory data should be obtained as close as possible to the time when fluids are to be assessed.

3. Determine (guess!) the expected change in weight over the monitoring period.

a. Given a 1,000-gm infant at birth, expected to lose about 15% of its birth weight, one might predict a 2% to 4% weight loss over the first 12 hours.

b. Given a 1,200-gm infant receiving 150 cc/kg/24 hr, but only given 40 calories/kg/24 hr, one might expect a calorie deficit of about 20 calories/kg/24 hr. Since the infant has little fat, the infant would need to burn 4 to 5 gm of protein to make up the calorie deficit and thus lose 4 to 5 gm in weight over 24 hours even though fluid intake was adequate.

4. Conditions that may alter fluid requirements are as follows:

a. Acute tubular necrosis (ATN) following asphyxia may produce oliguria.

b. Reduced GFR with hyaline membrane disease (HMD) or RDS decreases urine output.

c. Shock, pituitary, and renal dysfunction can all affect urine output.

d. Third spacing after bowel surgery.

e. Inappropriate anti-diuretic hormone secretion.

8

Nutrition

The goal of good nutrition is to provide sufficient calories and other nutrients to obtain optimal growth and development.

A. REQUIREMENTS

1. **Calories** Growth is dependent on intake beyond requirements for temperature control and physical activity (Table 8–1).

   a. In a neutral thermal environment with minimal physical work, caloric needs to maintain body weight are 50 to 60 kcal/kg/day (parenteral nutrition) or 60 to 75 kcal/kg/day (oral).

   b. Approximately 120 kcal/kg/day are required for sustained growth (15 to 30 gm weight per day).

TABLE 8–1.—DAILY CALORIC
EXPENDITURE IN A GROWING
PREMATURE INFANT*

ITEM	KCAL/KG/24 HR
Resting expenditure	40–50
Physical activity	15–30
Cold stress	10–70
Specific dynamic action	8
Fecal loss of calories	12
Growth allowance	25
Total	120

*Modified from Sinclair I.C., Driscoll J.M., Jr, Heird W.C., et al.: Supportive management of the sick neonate. *Pediatr. Clin. North Am.* 17:863, 1970.

2. Protein

a. Breast milk or a whey-predominant formula (whey:casein 60:40), which is higher in cysteine and lower in phenylalanine and tyrosine, is preferred.

   i. Premature infants have impaired metabolism of phenylalanine to tyrosine and tyrosine to homogentisic acid.

   ii. Generation of cysteine from methionine is impaired.

   iii. Bezoar formation from undigested casein is reduced.

b. Protein requirements are 2.2 to 3.5 gm/kg/day.

   i. Protein should constitute about 7% to 15% of the total caloric intake (4 kcal per gram of protein). Do not exceed 0.5 to 1.0 gm/kg/day until caloric intake exceeds 50 to 70 kcal/kg/day.

   ii. High protein intake may result in metabolic acidosis and elevated tyrosine, BUN, and ammonia levels (monitor BUN).

3. Fat

a. Thirty-five percent to 50% of total calories should be fat, i.e., 4 to 6 gm/kg/day (9 kcal/gm). Ketosis may occur if fat provides more than 60% of calories.

b. Long-chain fatty acids are inefficiently absorbed in small premature infants due to decreased intraluminal bile salts.

c. Medium-chain fatty acids and triglycerides (MCT) do not require micelle formation with bile salts for absorption.

4. Carbohydrate

a. Lactose intolerance is uncommon in the absence of gut injury even in premature infants less than 28 weeks' gestation.

b. Forty percent to 60% of total calories should be carbohydrates, i.e., 11 to 16 gm/kg/day (4 kcal/mg).

5. Vitamins

a. Requirements are not precisely known. Currently recommended daily intakes are listed in Table 8–2.

b. Multivitamins

   i. Adequate for infants with a daily intake of 800 to 1,000 ml/day of human milk or standard proprietary formulas.

   ii. Since premature infants do not consume this quantity, vitamin supplementation (e.g., Polyvisol®, 1 ml, diluted 1:3 with water or added to milk) should be given when

TABLE 8–2.—Suggested Daily Requirements
of Vitamins

VITAMIN	RECOMMENDED DAILY ORAL INTAKE*	POLYVISOL® (1 ML)
Vitamin A (IU)	500	1,500
Vitamin D (IU)	400 (800)	400
Vitamin E (IU)	4 (25)	5
Vitamin K (μg)	15	. . .
Vitamin C (mg)	20 (60)	35
Thiamin (mg)	0.2	0.5
Riboflavin (mg)	0.4	0.6
Pyridoxine (mg)	0.4	0.4
Niacin (mg)	5	8
Vitamin B (μg)	(1.5)	2
Folic acid (μg)	50 (60)	. . .

*Brackets indicate intake for premature infant, when different from term infant.

oral intake reaches about 80 kcal/kg/day. Similac Special Care® formula has adequate vitamins except for vitamin D.
  iii. All other "premature formulas" require multivitamins for supplementation.

c. Vitamin K
  i. At birth, administer 0.5 mg IM to infants weighing less than 1,500 gm, and 1.0 mg IM to infants weighing more than 1,500 gm.
  ii. Give vitamin K, 1 mg IM weekly, if infant is receiving total parenteral nutrition, or broad-spectrum antibiotics for more than ten days.

d. Vitamin E
  i. Body stores are very low at birth in the very small premature infant, and vitamin E is not well absorbed by the gut in these infants.
  ii. Vitamin E deficiency may result in hemolytic anemia, increased platelets, and edema. Hemolysis may be potentiated by increased intake of iron and polyunsaturated fatty acids.
  iii. We recommend that infants weighing less than 1,500 gm at birth receive 25 international units (IU) of vitamin E per day beginning on day 2 to 3 of life and continuing for six to eight weeks or until they reach 1,800 to 2,000 gm. The

solution (50 IU/ml) is hypertonic, and should be diluted or added to formula. We give 0.25 ml of Aquasol E®, diluted to 1.0 ml, twice daily.

e. Folic acid
   i. Folic acid levels are low in premature infants, and in certain other conditions (e.g., erythroblastosis fetalis).
   ii. Supplement with folacin, 50 μg/day orally or IV.

6. Minerals

a. Iron
   i. During the last trimester, the fetus accumulates 1.5 to 2.0 mg/kg/day. Therefore, prematurely born infants have minimal iron stores.
   ii. "Premature" formulas supply about 0.5 to 0.45 mg/kg/day when the infant is receiving 150 ml/kg/day. We recommend supplementing growing premature infants with iron (2 mg/kg/day) when they are 6 to 8 weeks old and continuing supplementation for three to four months, unless placed on iron-fortified formulas.

b. Calcium/phosphorus
   i. Fluctuations in serum calcium level in the first days of life reflect metabolic or hormonal adaptations. During this time, administration is indicated only to prevent or treat symptoms of serum hypocalcemia rather than to promote skeletal growth and mineralization.
   ii. The accumulation of calcium by the fetus during the last trimester averages 130 to 150 mg/kg/day. The calcium content of neither breast milk (35 mg/dl) nor standard infant formulas (55 mg/dl) is adequate to meet this accretion rate. "Premature" formulas contain 75 to 144 mg of calcium per deciliter.
   iii. Calcium absorption by the gut is inefficient (50% to 60% of intake), and calcium loss in urine is increased by diuretics, especially furosemide.
   iv. Very small premature infants are at risk for development of osteoporosis and poor linear growth.
   v. Calcium supplementation is recommended for infants weighing less than 1,000 gm if they are 2 weeks old, tolerating enteral feedings, but receiving less than 1,500 mg of calcium per kilogram per day (Table 8–3). Add 10% calcium gluconate (9 mg of calcium per milliliter) or calcium glubionate (23 mg of calcium per milliliter) to feedings to provide a total of 150 to 200 mg of calcium per kilogram per day until the infant weighs 1,500 to 2,000 gm.

TABLE 8–3.—Nutritional Supplementation of
Premature Infants (1,500 gm) Receiving Oral
Feeds

SUPPLEMENT	RECOMMENDATION
Polyvisol®, 1 ml	Start when oral intake reaches 80 kcal/kg/day
Vitamin E, 25 IU/day	Start day 2–3 of life if tolerated; continue 8 wk or until infant reaches 1,800–2,000 gm weight
Folate, 50 mcg/day	Start day 2–7 of life when oral intake tolerated; continue until infant reaches 1,800–2,000 gm
Iron, 2 mg/kg/day	Start at 6–8 wk, continue supplementation for 3–4 mo unless placed on iron-fortified formula
Calcium glubionate, 50–150 mg/kg/day (Neo-Calglucon syrup 23 mg/Ca/ml)	If enteral feeds are tolerated but do not provide 150 mg Ca/kg/day, supplement to provide daily calcium intake of 150–200 mg/kg/day. Divide dose in formula or breast milk. Continue until infant reaches 1,500–2,000 gm

*Note: Similac Special Care® formula has adequate vitamins
except for vitamin D. When using this formula supplement with
vitamin D (as D_3) 400 IU/day.

c. *Other elements* Breast milk and proprietary formulas provide quantities of magnesium, copper, zinc, manganese,
and iodine in excess of current recommendations for term
infants.

B. COMPOSITION OF MILK AND FORMULAS

1. **Commercially Prepared Formulas** generally attempt to
mimic human milk in terms of caloric density (67 kcal/dl or 20
kcal/oz) and distribution of calories between carbohydrate, fat,
and protein.

TABLE 8–4A.—Standard Infant Formulas

FORMULA	Kcal/ 100 ml	CARBOHYDRATE Gm/100 ml	FAT	PROTEIN
Milk				
Human Milk	68	7.1	4.5	1.1
Cow's Milk	68	4.8	3.7	3.3
Standard Formulas				
Similac with iron	68	7.2	3.6	1.5
Similac with whey/ iron	68	7.2	3.6	1.5
Enfamil with iron	68	6.9	3.8	1.5
SMA	68	7.2	3.6	1.5
Similac PM 60/40	68	6.9	3.8	1.5
Premature Formulas				
Similac Special Care (24)	81	8.6	4.4	2.2
Enfamil Premature (24)	81	8.9	4.1	2.4
SMA "Preemie" (24)	81	8.6	4.4	2.0
Special Formulas				
Isomil	68	6.8	3.6	2.0
Prosobee	68	6.9	3.6	2.0
Nutramigen	68	8.8	2.	2.2
Pregestimil	68	9.1	2.7	1.9

2. **Standard Infant Formulas** SMA®, and Similac PM 60:40®, Similac with whey, and Enfamil® contain a whey:casein ratio similar to human milk (60:40). Some standard formulas still contain protein with a ratio of whey to casein similar to cow's milk (18:82) (Table 8–4 A and B).

3. **"Premature" Formulas** contain a higher caloric density (81 kcal/dl or 24 kcal/oz), provide carbohydrates as a mixture of lactose and glucose polymers, provide higher levels of medium-chain triglycerides, electrolytes, calcium, and protein (whey:casein ratio of 60:40), minerals and vitamins.

CARBOHYDRATE COMPOSITION	FAT COMPOSITION	PROTEIN COMPOSITION OR WHEY : CASEIN RATIO
Lactose	Human Milk Fat	60:40
Lactose	Butterfat	18:82
Lactose	Soy, Coconut Oils	18:82
Lactose	Soy, Coconut Oils	60:40
Lactose	Soy, Coconut Oils	60:40
Lactose	Corn, Soy, Coconut Oils	60:40
Lactose	Corn, Coconut Oils	60:40
Lactose: Glucose Polymers = 50:50	MCT (50%), Corn, Coconut Oils	60:40
Lactose, Corn Syrup Solids	MCT (40%), Corn, Coconut Oils	60:40
Lactose: Glucose Polymers = 50:50	MCT (13%), Oleo, Oleic, Coconut, Soy Oils	60:40
Corn Syrup Solids, Sucrose	Soy, Coconut Oils	Soy Isolate Methionine
Corn Syrup Solids	Soy, Coconut Oils	Soy Isolate, Methionine
Sucrose, Tapioca Starch	Corn Oil	Casein Hydrolysate
Corn Syrup Solids Tapioca Starch	MCT, Corn Oil	Casein Hydrolysate

4. **Special Formulas** provide proteins as soy or casein hydrolysates, usually with a nonlactose source for carbohydrate.

C. POSTNATAL INTRODUCTION OF NUTRIENTS

1. **Tolerance to Fasting** is determined by the energy needs and energy reserves (Tables 8–1 and 8–5).

2. **SGA or Premature Infants** should receive IV glucose

TABLE 8–4B.—Standard Infant Formulas

FORMULA	Na mEq/L	K mEq/L	Ca mg/L	P mg/L	Ca/P	IRON mg/L	APPROX. RENAL mOsm/L	SOLUTE LOAD GI mOsm/L
Milk								
Human Milk	7–8	14–15	340	160	2.1	0.5	77	270
Cow Milk	25	35	1240	950	1.3	1.0	240	260
Standard Formulas								
Similac with iron	10	21	510	390	1.35	12	105	260
Similac with whey/iron	10	19	400	300	1.33	12	100	270
Enfamil with iron	9	18	460	320	1.46	12.7	100	270
SMA	7	14	440	330	1.33	12.7	92	270
Similac PM 60/40	7	15	400	200	2.0	1.5	96	240
Premature Formulas								
Similac Special Care (24)	17	29	1440	720	2.0	3.0	208	260
Enfamil Premature (24)	14	23	950	480	2.0	1.3	220	260
SMA "Preemie" (24)	14	19	750	400	1.9	3.0	175	240
Special Formulas								
Isomil	14	20	700	500	1.4	12	130	230
Prosobee	13	21	630	500	1.2	12.7	130	180
Nutramigen	14	17.5	630	475	1.33	12.7	130	430
Pregestimil	14	19	630	423	1.5	12.7	120	310

TABLE 8–5.—Estimated Energy Reserves

	SMALL PREMATURE		LARGE PREMATURE		TERM INFANT	
	GM	% BODY WEIGHT	GM	% BODY WEIGHT	GM	% BODY WEIGHT
Body weight	1,000		2,000		3,500	
Fat	10	1	100	5	560	16
Protein	85	8.5	230	11	390	11
Carbohydrate	4.5	0.5	9	0.5	34	1

(Adapted from Heird W.C., Driscoll J.M. Jr., Schullinger J.N., et al.: J. Pediatr. 80:351–372, 1972.)

by 4 to 6 hours of age if they cannot be fed orally. Infants with respiratory disease or feeding intolerance should receive supplemental protein/glucose by peripheral vein or central venous line starting day 3 to 6.

3. Factors Limiting Feeding Tolerance in Small Infants

a. Small stomach and delayed emptying.

b. Fat malabsorption, primarily due to low concentrations of bile salts.

c. Intolerance to high osmotic load, producing abdominal distention, GI tract bleeding, necrotizing enterocolitis.

d. May be intolerant to formulas with high casein content due to large curd formation, higher phenylalanine, or tyrosine load.

4. Mode of Feedings Route selected depends on gestational age, illness, and vigor (nipple or breast, gavage, nasojejunal tube).

a. Most infants under 32 to 33 weeks' gestation nipple poorly, have immature gag and swallowing reflexes, and require gavage feeding.

b. Some small premature infants (<1,000 gm) tolerate continuous feedings (by pump) through a nasogastric tube or nasojejunal tube when intermittent gavage is not tolerated.
   i. *Nasogastric tube:* A No. 5 French polyethylene tube is used and changed every 12 hours. Check for gastric residuals before each feeding.
   ii. *Nasojejunal tube:* A mercury-tipped silastic tube should be used. Polyethylene tubes may harden and cause intestinal perforation. Place the infant on the right side to facilitate passage through the pylorus. Proper positioning is suspected by return of bile, or a pH reading on the aspirate greater than 5. Confirm roentgenographically. Several hours may be required for passage of the tube.

5. The material fed sick premature infants usually progresses from sterile water to 13-calorie formula or breast milk, 20 calories per ounce of formula, to 24 calories per ounce of premature formula. Near-term infants can usually be advanced to full-strength formula after an initial water feeding.

a. Breast milk can be expressed by mother and given by gavage to infants if they cannot suckle. Breast milk may be an inadequate single source of nutrition for the very small premature infant, and he or she may require supplementation with protein, vitamins, electrolytes, and calories.

b. Selection of formula should consider osmolality and renal solute load (see Table 8–4 B). Limited ability to concentrate or dilute urine makes the premature infant vulnerable to high solute load or excessive insensible water loss.

c. "Premature formulas" are designed to meet the needs of the growing premature infant weighing less than 1,800 to 2,000 gm.

d. Special formulas may be required for infants with cardiac, electrolyte, or digestive disorders.

6. **Use of Caloric Supplements** when an infant requires fluid restriction or is not growing on 120 kcal/kg/day is as follows:

a. High caloric formulas with inadequate free water may provide too high a renal solute load resulting in hyperosmolality and hypernatremia.

b. Medium-chain triglycerides
   i. If added to formula, do not exceed 60% of total calories as fat.
   ii. 24 kcal per ounce of formula plus 0.4 ml of MCT oil per ounce provides 27 kcal per ounce of formula.

c. Glucose polymers (Polycose®, Ross Laboratory)
   i. It is generally preferable to increase fat before supplementing with carbohydrate.
   ii. 27 kcal per ounce of formula plus 1.5 cc of Polycose per ounce provides 30 kcal per ounce of formula.

7. **Frequency of Feeding** Small premature infants are usually started on two-hour feedings, increasing to every three hours. Babies should be on three- to four-hour interval feeds before discharge.

8. **Amount of Feeding**

a. Start small infants on sterile water, 2 to 3 ml/kg for one to three feedings. Then start half strength or 13 calorie/ounce of formula.

b. Increase volume 1 to 2 ml every two to four feedings as tolerated.

c. Increase caloric strength as tolerated when about 50% fluids are taken by mouth.

    d. Larger premature and term infants are started on 5 to 10 ml/kg feedings and advanced more rapidly.

    e. Intolerance to feeding may require temporary cessation of feeding and assessment of the patient.

9. **Tolerance to Oral Feeding** is judged by the following:

    a. Stomach residuals obtained before each feeding; these should be less than 3 ml or 30% of volume, whichever is larger.

    b. Vomiting or regurgitation of formula.

    c. Abdominal distention.

    d. Heme or sugar present in stool.

D. MONITORING SUCCESS

1. Careful weekly measurement of head circumference and length with plotting on a growth graph is important.

2. Daily weights are plotted on growth graph chart, and trends as well as day-to-day changes must be assessed.

REFERENCES

1. Committee on Nutrition, American Academy of Pediatrics: Nutritional needs of low-birth-weight infants. *Pediatrics* 60:519–530, 1977.
2. Ziegler E.E., Biga R.L., Fomon S.J.: Nutritional requirements of the premature infant, in Suskind R.M. (ed): *Textbook of Pediatric Nutrition.* New York, Raven Press, 1981.

9

Parenteral Nutrition

Parenteral nutrition (PN) refers to the IV administration of amino acids, carbohydrates, and fats together with minerals, vitamins, and trace metals. Small premature infants have little energy reserves as seen by the calculated tolerance to malnourishment in newborns and adults (Table 9–1).

A. INDICATIONS FOR PARENTERAL NUTRITION

1. Premature neonate (<1,500 gm) in whom the combined oral and IV caloric intake is anticipated to be less than 90 calories/kg by 1 week of age.

2. Any infant over 1 week of age who does not receive more than 80 to 90 calories/kg by combined oral and IV routes.

B. ROUTE OF ADMINISTRATION

1. Central Vein

a. Silastic Broviac catheters. These are radiopaque infant Bro-

TABLE 9–1.—CALCULATED SURVIVAL TIME IN DAYS IN STARVATION AND SEMISTARVATION

	WATER ONLY*	10% DEXTROSE
Small premature infant	4	11
Large premature infant	12	30
Full-term infant	33	80
Adult	90	350

*Seventy-five milliliters per kilogram per day for infant; 3 L/day for adult. (Adapted from Heird W.C., Driscoll J.M., Schullinger J.N., et al.: *J. Pediatr.* 80:351, 1970.

viac catheters, 1.3 mm outer diameter, placed by the pediatric surgeon.

   i. Following a cutdown over the common facial vein, the catheter is threaded into the internal jugular vein, and into the superior vena cava. Placement is verified with x-ray.
   ii. Complication rate is high in very small infants, and the fine silastic catheters, introduced percutaneously or by cutdown, are preferred to the infant Broviac catheters in neonates weighing less than 1,000 gm.

   b. Peripherally introduced central fine silastic catheters are generally preferred for total PN (TPN) administration.

2. **Peripheral Vein** Scalp vein needles and angiocaths are used for peripheral PN. Glucose concentrations should not exceed 12.5 mg/dl. Care should be taken if large amounts of calcium are being administered (>100 mg/dl IV solutions).

3. **Umbilical Artery Catheter (UAC)** is not used for PN in our nursery unless approved by the attending neonatologist. This route is only used temporarily for infants weighing less than 750 gm.

C. CATHETER CARE

1. Fine silastic deep lines and Broviac catheters are maintained by the nursing staff and TPN nursing team. No central PN line should be entered unless using aseptic technique. No central line is to be used for blood drawing, infusion products, or medications except in emergencies.

2. Broviac catheter sites are covered with gauze sponge and a small amount of povidone-iodine (Betadine) ointment, changed daily.

3. Fine silastic deep lines should be maintained with a dry dressing, if collodion is used as a stabilizer.

4. Peripheral lines should be treated in a similar fashion as central lines.

5. Lipids (e.g., Intralipid®) may be infused simultaneously with amino acid solutions by using a "Y" connector attached to the PN catheter. A Millipore filter (0.22 μ filter unit) is attached to the "Y" connector arm leading to amino acid solutions. Lipids are administered unfiltered through the second arm.

TABLE 9-2.—Guidelines for Glucose, Amino Acid, and Lipid Infusion

	STARTING AMOUNT	MAXIMUM AMOUNT	DAYS TO ATTAIN MAXIMUM	LABORATORY MONITORING	MAXIMUM CALORIES
Glucose	11 gm/kg*	20 gm/kg	6–12 days†	Urine-serum glucose, Dextrostix	80 calories/kg
Amino acids	0.5 gm/kg	2.5 gm/kg	5–10 days	Total protein NH₃, BUN, creatinine, pH, liver enzymes, bilirubin‡	10 calories/kg
Lipid	0.5 gm/kg	4 gm/kg	8–16 days	Serum turbidity; triglycerides orally with lung disease	44 calories/kg

*May need to start lower if glucose intolerant.
†May take longer if glucose intolerant.
‡NH₃ indicates ammonia; BUN, blood urea nitrogen.

D. SOLUTION GUIDELINES (Table 9–2)   Standardized solutions are not used in our nursery. (See special order sheet, Figure 9–1.)

1. Glucose

a. Infusion generally begins at 4 to 6 mg/kg/min and is increased by 0.5 to 1.2 mg/kg/min (or approximately 1.0 to 2.0 gm/kg/day) every day as tolerated. Most infants do not tolerate more than 12 to 15 mg/kg/min.

b. Dextrostix® readings are obtained at least every 12 hours

UNIVERSITY OF CALIFORNIA - DAVIS
MEDICAL CENTER
SACRAMENTO
PHYSICIANS ORDERS
NICU PARENTERAL NUTRITION

PATIENT Wt.:_____ kg

	DATE	HOUR	USE BALL POINT PEN					USE PATIENT DATA PLATE
	DATE	HOUR	AMOUNT PT. TO RECV/DAY	TOTAL AMOUNT ml PREP/DAY ml	TO RUN AT ml/hr		Refer to Instruction#	
					Estimated Req/24 Hours			
			AMINO ACID _____ Gm	_____ Gm	0.5Gm-2.5Gm Protein/kg (provides 0.4mEq Cl & 0.9mEq Ac/Gm)		#2	
			DEXTROSE _____ Gm	_____ Gm	7-20 Gm Dextrose/kg		#1	
			NaCl _____ mEq	_____ mEq	3-6 mEq Na/Kg		#3	
			* K Phosphate _____ mM (4.4mEq K AND 3mM PO₄/ml)	_____ mM	0.5-1mM PO₄/kg (Provides 0.75-1.45mEq K/kg of the total daily req.)		#4,5	
			* K Acetate _____ mEq	_____ mEq	2-4mEq K/kg		#5,6	
			MgSO₄ _____ mEq	_____ mEq	0.25 mEq Mg/kg			
			Ca Gluc _____ mEq	_____ mEq	0.25-0.75mEq Ca/kg		#7	
			MVI CONC _____ ml	_____ ml	1ml MVI CONC		#10	
			Folic Acid _____ mg	_____ mg	0.05mg Folic Acid/kg			
			B12 _____ mcg	_____ mcg	5mcg B12/kg			
			Zn SO₄ _____ mg	_____ mg	0.3mg Zn/kg		#8	
			Cu SO₄ _____ mg	_____ mg	0.03mg Cu/Kg		#9	
			HEPARIN _____ Units	_____ Units	1/2 Unit/ml			
			* * * * * * * * *					
			NICU INTRALIPID ORDER					
			INTRALIPID 10% _____ ml/hr x _____ hrs. daily 0.2-4Gm/kg/day				#11	
			ROUTE OF ADMINISTRATION: CENTRAL _____ PERIPHERAL _____					
			PHYSICIAN SIGNATURE:					

Fig 9–1.—Calculation and order form for parenteral nutrition solutions.

and more often if changes are made, or the infant's glucose level is elevated. If the Dextrostix reading or serum glucose level is greater than 130 mg/dl or urine glucose level is greater than 2+, then glucose concentration must be decreased.

   c. Insulin (0.25 to 0.5 units/kg) may be necessary if lowering the glucose concentration is not effective.

2. Amino Acids

   a. Begin at 0.5 gm/kg and increase by 0.25 to 0.5 gm/kg/day to a maximum of 2.5 gm/kg/day.

   b. Ratio of nonprotein-to-protein calories should be approximately 10:1.

   c. Total protein, ammonia (NH_3), BUN, serum creatinine, serum pH, liver enzyme, and bilirubin values and urine output should be monitored.

   d. The contents of amino acid solutions vary by manufacturer. Both FreAmine III® 10% and Travasol®10% are acceptable solutions for neonates and contain the percentages of essential amino acids required by these infants.
      i. Arginine is present in sufficient quantities to reduce the incidence of hyperammonemia.
      ii. Chloride contents are low, an important consideration with respect to metabolic acidosis. Travasol 10% contains 0.4 mEq of chloride and 0.9 mEq of acetate per gram of amino acid, and FreAmine III 10% contains significant amounts of chloride and 0.7 mEq of acetate per gram of amino acid.
      iii. Branched-chain amino acid (BCAA) as compared with other solutions—BCAAs are anticatabolic and provide the substrate to meet the necessary energy requirements that occur during stress and sepsis.

3. Lipid

   a. Intralipid® infusion is begun at 0.5 gm/kg/day and increased to 4 gm/kg/day in increments of 0.25 to 0.5 gm/kg/day. The infusion rate should not exceed 1.6 ml/kg/hr (10% emulsion) in preterm infants (<33 weeks) and no more than 3 ml/kg/hr in infants greater than 33 weeks' gestation.

   b. Serum turbidity should be monitored by nephelometry or visually, two to eight hours after an infusion. If serum is turbid, then the amount of Intralipid should be decreased or the infusion time lengthened. Serum triglyceride levels should be measured once a week.

c. Calories from fat should not exceed 45% of the total daily caloric intake.

d. Risk for bacterial and fungal growth increases when a lipid bottle is open longer than 12 hours. When it is not possible to infuse a daily requirement in 12 hours or less, then two 30-ml bottles should be ordered and changed after 12 hours.

e. There should be at least four to eight hours of noninfusion time daily for serum clearing of Intralipid.

E. SPECIAL CONSIDERATIONS

1. **Fluid, Electrolyte, or Metabolic Imbalance** may necessitate temporary (e.g., 24 hours) discontinuation of PN.

2. **Renal Failure** may necessitate limiting amino acid administration to 0.5 to 1.0 gm/kg/day. Use the BUN concentration as a guide.

3. **Hepatic Failure** Amino acid administration to an infant with hepatic insufficiency may result in serum amino acid imbalances, azotemia, and hyperammonemia. Discontinue PN if liver enzymes are markedly elevated in serum.

4. **Central Venous Lines for PN** should not be placed when sepsis or suspected sepsis is present until the blood is sterilized. Parenteral nutrition during this time can be administered by a peripheral vein with appropriate considerations of solution osmolality, calcium content, etc.

F. COMPLICATIONS

1. **Infiltration of PN Solutions in Peripheral Veins** may cause local subcutaneous tissue injury and skin sloughs.

2. **Metabolic**

a. *Hypoglycemia* Discontinuation of IV solutions in infants receiving PN may cause the glucose level to fall rapidly. Therefore, the infusion must be restarted as soon as possible. If the daily infusion falls behind the expected rate, any effort to catch up must be done gradually over eight to 24 hours without exceeding the infant's ability to tolerate glucose.

b. *Hyperglycemia* Glucose administration is increased gradually to avoid hyperglycemia. Glycosuria may accompany hyperglycemia and lead to serious dehydration.

c. *Hyperammonemia* is due to excessive amino acid administration. Decreasing or temporarily discontinuing protein administration will correct this problem. This occurs infrequently, since arginine in PN solutions has been increased. Ammonia levels should be monitored weekly.

d. *Hyperlipidemia* SGA infants are particularly prone to hyperlipidemia. Intralipid should be used with caution in infants with lung disease. If increasing supplemental oxygen is required with no apparent cause, consideration should be given to decreasing or temporarily discontinuing Intralipid administration.

e. *Fluid or electrolyte imbalance* The infant's fluid and electrolyte status should be evaluated before ordering new solutions.

f. *Metabolic acidosis* is usually induced by hyperchloremia. It may be necessary to give more anions as acetate. The dose of amino acids should be checked. Sepsis must be ruled out.

g. *Liver damage* Progressive cholestasis, with direct hyperbilirubinemia, portal tract fibrosis, and infiltration occur with prolonged amino acid administration. Liver function returns to normal one to four months after discontinuation of PN.

3. Infection (sepsis)

a. Catheters for parenteral nutrition should be removed if blood cannot be sterilized after 48 hours of appropriate antibiotic therapy. Catheters should be removed immediately if the infant clinically deteriorates.

b. Mechanical (notify attending physician, fellow)
   i. Catheter leakage
   ii. Catheter clotting
   iii. Catheter breakage
   iv. Venous thrombosis
   v. Hydrothorax

G. MONITORING INFANTS

1. Clinical

a. Weigh—usually once a shift (depends on age and size of patient and duration of therapy).

TABLE 9–3.—LABORATORY TESTS FOR MONITORING INFANTS RECEIVING PN*

TEST	SUGGESTED FREQUENCY
Urine specific gravity, Glucose, protein pH (done in the nursery)	Each shift until stable and gaining weight, then once a week
Dextrostix® (done in nursery)	Every 12 hours and more often if changes are made or glucose level is elevated
Hematocrit	2–3 times per week
CBC, platelets with differential	2–3 times per week
CBG or ABG	1–3 times per week (unless receiving blood gas monitoring for respiratory disease)
Na, K, Cl, Ca, BUN	Daily first week, then 2 times a week when stable. Included in Chem 20 once a week
Total/direct bilirubin	2 times a week, or more often if indicated
Serum and urine osmolality	Once a week
Magnesium	Once a week
Twenty-factor automated chemical analysis, particularly for SGOT, SGPT, albumin, phosphate, creatine, total protein, triglycerides	Once a week
NH_3	Once a week
Glucose	Daily first week and if glycosuria 2 + and/or Dextrostix >130
Serum turbidity	Daily first week, 2–8 hours after Intralipid infusion (If turbid, measure triglyceride level, decrease dose or lengthen infusion time)

*PN indicates parenteral nutrition; CBC, complete blood cell count; CBG, capillary blood gas; ABG, arterial blood gas; Na, sodium; K, potassium; Cl, chlorine; Ca, calcium; BUN, blood urea nitrogen; SGOT, serum glutamic ox-aloacetic transaminase; SGPT, serum glutamic-pyruvic transaminase; NH_3, ammonia.

b. Intake and output.

c. Head circumference—daily.

d. Liver size (palpation by physician daily).

2. Laboratory   Table 9–3.

REFERENCE

1. Shaw J.C.L.: Parenteral nutrition in the management of sick low-birth-weight infants. *Pediatr. Clinics* 20:333, 1973.

10

Infections

I. INFECTIONS OF MATERNAL ORIGIN

The list (Table 10–1) of agents transmissible from the mother to the fetus and neonate includes more than the traditional TORCH agents (toxoplasmosis, other [syphilis], rubella, cytomegalovirus, and herpes). Some prenatal infections result in the typical TORCH syndrome of hepatosplenomegaly, jaundice, purpura, CNS signs, and intrauterine growth retardation. Most newborns experiencing prenatal infection are asymptomatic. The various infections are often clinically indistinguishable from one another. The diagnosis is based on several methods:

1. Detection and isolation of infectious agent.

   a. Electron microscopy (EM), immunofluorescence, cytologic findings.

   b. Immunodiffusion, counterimmunoelectrophoresis (CIE), enzyme-linked immunosorbant assay (ELISA).

   c. Culture (most reliable).

2. Persistence of specific IgG antibody beyond the age of normal decline of maternal antibody (three to four months).

3. *Total* IgM greater than 20 mg/dl only *suggests* intrauterine infection, but is nonspecific with both false-positive and false-negative results.

4. Elevation of IgM-*specific* antibody in cord or neonatal blood is significant, but some infants with intrauterine infection do not have IgM-specific antibody.

II. BACTERIAL INFECTIONS

Bacterial illnesses commonly encountered in the newborn include sepsis, meningitis, pneumonia, cutaneous infection, conjunctivitis,

TABLE 10–1.—Infectious Agents Transmissible From Mother to Infant

| | ONSET OF INFECTION | | TORCH SYNDROME | DIAGNOSTIC METHODS* |
	FETAL	PERINATAL		
Toxoplasma gondii	+	...	+	1, 2, 8, 9
Treponema Pallidum	+	...	+	2, 8, 10
Rubella	+	...	+	1, 8, 9
Cytomegalovirus	+	+	+	1, 2, 3, 8
Herpes simplex	+	+	+	1, 2, 3, 4
Hepatitis A	?	?	...	8
Hepatitis B	(rare)	+	...	10
Measles	+	+	?	1, 2, 9
Varicella	+	+	+	1, 2, 3, 4
Enterovirus	+	+	+	1, 9, 7
Malaria	...	...	...	2, 9
Tuberculosis	+	+	...	1, 2, 4
Chlamydia	...	...	...	1, 2, 8
GC	...	...	...	1
Listeria	+	+	+	1, 2, 9
Enteric bacteria	...	+	...	1
Hemophilus influenzae	...	+	...	1
Group B β hemolytic streptococcus	...	+	...	1, 5, 6
Candida albicans	(rare)	+	...	1, 2

*The most significant diagnostic tests are depicted by the larger figures. 1 indicates culture; 2, cytology; 3, EM; 4, immunofluorescence; 5, latex agglutination; 6, counterimmunoelectrophoresis; 7, ELISA; 8, IgM-specific antibody; 9, acute and convalescent specific IgG titer; 10, other serologic test or procedure.

urinary tract infection, and, less commonly, arthritis and osteomyelitis.

A. SIGNS AND SYMPTOMS

These are variable and often nonspecific. Sepsis simulates many noninfectious conditions. Temperature instability with hypothermia or hyperthermia may be present. Additional signs may include poor sucking, vomiting, diarrhea, abdominal distention, apnea, respiratory distress, cyanosis, hepatosplenomegaly, jaundice, skin mottling, lethargy, hypotonia, and seizures. Bulging fontanel and nuchal rigidity are not reliable signs of meningitis in the newborn.

B. "SEPSIS WORK-UP"

1. **Culture** Blood, cerebrospinal fluid (CSF), urine, tracheal secretions, and obvious sites of infection.

2. **Gram's Stain** Buffy coat, CSF, urine, tracheal secretions, and infected sites.

3. **CSF** Culture, Gram's stain, cell count, protein, glucose.

   a. Normal CSF findings in high-risk newborns are shown in Table 10–2.

   b. Cloudy CSF may result from bacterial proliferation in the absence of pleocytosis. Less than 1% of infants with meningitis will have a totally normal initial lumbar puncture, although glucose/protein responses may be minimal.

   c. Low blood glucose level and polymorphonuclear response may occur with intraventricular hemorrhage.

   d. Ventricular tap may be necessary to document ventriculitis in patients with hydrocephalus (e.g., meningomyelocele).

4. **Tracheal Aspirate** In the immediate neonatal period, leukocytes and bacteria on Gram's stain suggest congenital infection.

5. **White Blood Cell (WBC), Differential, and Platelet Count** Normal WBC and differential counts do not rule out sepsis. Leukopenia and neutropenia or an increase in the total band count, with ratio of bands to total neutrophils 0.2

TABLE 10–2.—NORMAL CSF FINDINGS
IN HIGH-RISK NEWBORNS*

RANGE	TERM INFANT	PRETERM INFANT
WBC count (cells/cu mm)	0–32	0–29
% PMNs†	~60%	~60%
Protein, mg/dl	20–170	65–150
Glucose, mg/dl	34–119	24–63
CSF/blood glucose, %	44–248	55–105

*Adapted from Sarff LD et al. (*J. Pediatr.* 88:473, 1976).
†PMN indicates polymorphonuclear neutrophil leukocytes.

or greater, suggest sepsis but may be present in nonseptic stressed premature infants. Thrombocytopenia occurs in sepsis with or without disseminated intravascular clotting (DIC).

6. **Chest X-ray** Pneumonia may look like HMD, wet lung, or pneumonia.

7. **Suprapubic Aspiration or Bladder Catheterization**

   a. *Urine culture* On suprapubic aspirate cultures, any number of a single bacterium is considered significant. A bagged urine culture is useful when sterile (uncommon); recovery of more than 100,000 single or mixed flora requires repeated culture by suprapubic aspirate to confirm.

   b. *Urinalysis* Pyuria may accompany urinary tract infection (UTI), but false-positive and false-negative results are encountered. Finding more than 5 bacteria per high-power field (hpf) on Gram's stain of unspun urine indicates infection.

8. **Erythrocyte Sedimentation Rate (ESR)** Capillary blood in a 75-mm heparinized microhematocrit tube, ESR 15 mm/hr or higher in septic infants; infants with DIC and sepsis have low ESR. Normal values are age dependent: range, 1 mm/hr at 12 hours to 17 mm/hr at 14 days.

9. **Limulus Lysate Assay for Endotoxin Detection** is useful for detecting coliform sepsis and necrotizing enterocolitis (NEC) beyond the first week of life; not specific for bacteremia during the first week of life.[8]

10. **Latex Agglutination Test**, CIE identify bacterial antigens in serum, urine, or CSF. Detectable neonatal infections include group β streptococcus, *Hemophilus influenzae* B, certain serotypes of streptococcal pneumonia, and meningococci.

C. MANAGEMENT

1. **When Sepsis Is Suspected** obtain appropriate cultures and begin treatment with a combination of ampicillin and an aminoglycoside for three days or until sensitivity studies are completed on a recovered bacterium. Add an antistaphylococcal antimicrobic if *S. aureus* is suspected.

2. Duration of Treatment

a. *Sepsis without focal involvement* seven to ten days.

b. *Meningitis* 14 days after sterile CSF cultures are noted.

c. *Pneumonia* ten to 14 days for group B streptococcus and usual enterics; up to four weeks for *S. aureus.*

d. *UTI* Usually ten to 14 days.

3. Meningitis

a. Antibiotic choice should consider ability of the antimicrobic to achieve sustained bactericidal levels in the CSF.
   i. Chloramphenicol diffuses well into the CSF if the organism is sensitive.
   ii. Addition of third-generation cephalosporins, e.g., cefotaxime or moxalactam, may be effective when the initial CSF gram's stain shows gram-negative organisms. May be added to or substituted for gentamicin in the initial regimen.

b. Intrathecal administration of aminoglycoside is not effective. Intraventricular instillation of aminoglycoside has been associated with greater mortality and morbidity, but may be indicated in patients with meningomyeloceles depending on susceptibility of the organism.

4. Urinary Tract Infection

a. Repeat urine culture 48 to 72 hours after treatment is initiated, two weeks after treatment is completed, and at regular intervals for at least one year after infection.

b. Evaluate renal function (creatinine, BUN, etc.)

c. Intravenous pyelogram and voiding cystourethrogram are usually indicated to evaluate anatomic abnormalities, although neonatal infection may occur with normal urinary tract.

5. Additional Potentially Useful Maneuvers in Overwhelming Sepsis

a. *Exchange transfusion* Efficacy is not established. In group B β streptococcus sepsis, exchange transfusions with blood containing specific antibodies improved outcome.

b. *Granulocyte transfusion* Septic infants with neutropenia and depleted neutrophil marrow reserves may have improved survival following granulocyte transfusion.

D. CUTANEOUS INFECTION Pustules, impetigo, cellulitis, abscess.

1. **Etiology** varies with nature of skin lesion (Table 10–3). Certain skin lesions suggest particular infections, e.g., bullous lesions and *Treponema pallidum*, ecthyma gangrenosum, and *Pseudomonas aeruginosa*. The possibility of herpes simplex infection should be considered in vesicular-pustular lesions. Tender, erythematous, weeping desquamation of skin suggests staphylococcal scalded-skin syndrome. Erythema toxicum may sometimes mimic bacterial infection; scrapings show eosinophils and the absence of organisms.

2. **Diagnosis** Culture and gram-stain lesions, aspirate margin of cellulitis, scrape base of vesicular lesions for Tzanck preparation looking for multinucleated giant cells characteristic of herpes.

3. **Management** Limited superficial pustules usually require local topical treatment only. Extensive pustules, involvement of compromised skin sites, or both require systemic treatment with appropriate antimicrobics based on Gram's stain of the lesion, usually for seven to ten days.

E. CONJUNCTIVITIS (Table 10–4) Frequently bacterial; rare but important nonbacterial cause is herpes simplex

TABLE 10–3.—BACTERIAL CAUSES OF SKIN
LESIONS IN NEONATES

TYPE OF LESION	LIKELY CAUSE
Pustular-vesicular	*Staphylococcus aureus;* β strep; other bacteria and candida are less common
Cellulitis	Groups A and B β strep, *S. aureus,* gram-negative enterics
Abscess	*S. aureus;* Group B β strep, gram-negative enterics
Omphalitis	*S. aureus;* Group B β strep, gram-negative enterics
Scalded skin syndrome (Ritter's disease)	*S. aureus*

TABLE 10–4.—Conjunctivitis in the Neonate

TIME OF ONSET	LIKELY CAUSE	ORDER OF FREQUENCY OF INFECTION
12–24 hr (typically improving in 24 hr)	Chemical conjunctivitis (AgNO₃)	. . .
2–5 days	*Neisseria gonorrhoeae*	2
5–26 days	*Chlamydia trachomatis*	1 most common
1st week–1 month	*Staphylococcus aureus, gram-negative enterics; other bacteria*	3
Few days–few weeks	Herpes simplex	4

virus; a plugged nasolacrimal duct may be considered in older infants.

1. Diagnosis

a. Gram's stain and culture discharge.

b. Giemsa's stain of conjunctival scrapings detects intracytoplasmic inclusions of chlamydial infection.

c. Consider viral culture and Tzanck smear to look for multinucleated giant cells typical of herpes infection, if results of (a) and (b) above are negative.

2. Management and Treatment depend on origin of conjunctivitis.

a. *Chemical conjunctivitis*   No treatment indicated.

b. *Bacterial conjunctivitis* (other than gonorrheal) Topical—antimicrobics such as polymyxin-bactracin combinations, sulfa, erythromycin, or tetracycline are usually sufficient.

c. *Gonorrheal conjunctivitis*   Parenteral penicillin, 50,000 U/kg/day every 12 hours for seven to ten days, should be given in addition to topical treatment with erythromycin or tetracycline every two hours. The latter should be preceded by saline irrigations.

d. *Chlamydial conjunctivitis*   Topical treatment with sulfa or erythromycin applied four times a day for two to three weeks. Topical treatment does not effect later onset of chlamydial pneumonia. Oral erythromycin prevents onset of chlamydial pneumonia and suffices for treatment of chlamydial conjunctivitis.

e. *Pseudomonas conjunctivitis*   may cause particularly virulent infection and requires treatment with parenteral gentamicin or tobramycin plus ticarcillin in addition to topical aminoglycoside therapy.

F. ARTHRITIS AND OSTEOMYELITIS

Most episodes arise from bacteremic spread, but occasionally result from local extension or direct inoculation. Neonatal osteomyelitis may produce adjacent joint involvement.

1. Etiology includes *S. aureus,* group B β streptococcus, various gram-negative enterics, *Neisseria gonorrhoeae,* and *Candida.*

2. **Signs and Symptoms** often are unimpressive. Failure to move extremity or pain on movement may be noted by nursing personnel or caretaker. Swelling, erythema, and increased warmth are occasionally present.

3. Diagnostic Tests

a. X-ray film of joint, bone; repeat after ten days; roentgenographic findings in oxteomyelitis are negative early.

b. Bone scan is of limited usefulness in the neonate; it should be done, but many false-negative findings occur.

c. Blood culture.

d. Bone and joint aspiration for Gram's stain and culture.

4. Management

a. Nafcillin plus gentamicin are reasonable choices when the cause is unknown. Definitive treatment is based on results of culture and sensitivity. Intra-articular or intraosseous antimicrobics are unnecessary.

b. Duration or antimicrobic treatment depends on the nature of the infection.
   i. About two to three weeks for arthritis, about four to six weeks for osteomyelitis.
   ii. Oral antimicrobics should not be considered unless monitoring of serum bactericidal levels can be accomplished and compliance with treatment can be assured.
   iii. The ESR is a useful guide to duration of treatment. X-ray resolution of osteomyelitis is not a useful guide.

c. Surgical treatment
   i. Open drainage of hip is always indicated to prevent ischemia, necrosis, and permanent damage to femoral head and joint.
   ii. Other joints may be managed by repeated aspiration.
   iii. Bone infection should be surgically drained if pus is recovered from needle aspiration.

REFERENCES

1. Remington, J.A., Klein J. (eds.): *Infectious Diseases of the Fetus and Newborn.* Philadelphia, W.B. Saunders Co., 1983.
2. Feigen R.D., Cherry J.D. (eds.): *Textbook of Pediatric Infectious Diseases.* Philadelphia, W.B. Saunders Co., 1981.
3. Sherman, M.P., Goetzman B.W., Ahlfors C.E., et al.: Tracheal aspiration and its clinical correlates in diagnosis of congenital pneumonia. *Pediatrics* 65:258–263, 1980.

4. Monroe B.L.: The differential leukocyte count in the assessment and outcome of early onset neonatal group B streptococcal infection. *J. Pediatr.* 91:632, 1977.
5. Adler S.M., Denton R.L.: The erythrocyte sedimentation rate in the newborn period. *J. Pediatr.* 942–948, 1975.
6. Scheifele D.W., Melton P., Ebelt V.: Evaluation of Limulus test for endotoxemia in neonates with suspected sepsis. *J. Pediatr.* 98:899–903, 1981.
7. Vaine N.E., Mazlumian J.R., Swarner, O.W., et al.: Role of exchange transfusion in treatment of severe septicemia. *Pediatrics* 66:693, 1980.
8. Christensen R.D.: Granulocyte transfusions in neonates with bacterial infection, neutropenia and depletion of mature marrow neutrophils. *Pediatrics* 70:1, 1982.
9. McCracken G.H. Jr., Mize S.G., Threlkeld N.: Intraventricular gentamicin therapy in gram-negative bacillary meningitis of infancy. *Lancet* 1:787–791, 1980.
10. Swartz M.N.: Intraventricular use of aminoglycosides in treatment of gram-negative bacillary meningitis: Conflicting views. *J. Infect. Dis.* 143:293–296, 1981.

III. SPECIFIC BACTERIAL INFECTIONS

A. SYPHILIS

Treponema pallidum spirochetal infection. The spectrum of infection varies from asymptomatic infection to serious multiorgan involvement. Clinical signs include rhinitis, rash, hepatosplenomegaly, jaundice, lymphadenopathy, nephrosis, pseudoparalysis, stillbirth, prematurity, failure to thrive, and unexplained hydrops fetalis.

1. Diagnosis

a. Serological testing is the mainstay of diagnosis of syphilis.
   i. Screening tests for possible syphilis include so-called reagin (nonspecific) tests, e.g., VDRL, rapid plasma reagin (RPR), Kolmer, Hinton, and Kahn tests.
   ii. To establish the presence of syphilitic infection, these positive screening tests must be confirmed with a positive result to a specific treponemal test such as the fluorescent treponemal antibody-absorption test (FTA-ABS).
   iii. A positive FTA-ABS test in the neonate might represent transplacental transport of maternal IgG. The IgM FTA-ABS test, developed to confirm congenital neonatal syphilis infection, may not be reliable.

iv. While theoretically an ideal test for distinguishing infants with true congenital syphilis from infants who are FTA-ABS positive based solely on transplacental transmission of maternal IgG antibody, the test result is potentially unreliable. Thus, infants with a negative IgM-FTA-ABS finding should be followed with serial VDRL testing to confirm loss of serological reactivity.

b. Dark field examination of appropriate lesions for spirochetes, e.g., nasal discharge.

c. Pathologic examination of placenta.

d. X-ray film of long bones to look for syphilitic changes; osteochondritis, periostitis, and osteomyelitis.

e. Lumbar puncture to exclude asymptomatic neurosyphilis.

f. A CBC count with differential; monocytosis occurs in infants with symptomatic congenital syphilis.

2. **Management**   The appropriate management of syphilis in the neonate involves consideration of history, prior antimicrobic therapy of mother, and the clinical and serological status of mother and infant (Table 10–5).

a. If CSF is normal treat infant with penicillin G benzathine, 50,000 U/kg IM once.

b. If CSF is abnormal treat infant with the following:
   i. Penicillin G crystalline, 25,000 U/kg IM or IV twice a day for ten days, or
   ii. Penicillin G procaine, 50,000 U/kg IM daily for ten days.

B. GROUP B β-HEMOLYTIC STREPTOCOCCUS (GBS)   GBS causes a variety of neonatal infections including sepsis, pneumonia, meningitis, empyema, cellulitis, arthritis, osteomyelitis, and impetigo. Two clinically and epidemiologically distinct forms of GBS sepsis are described (Table 10–6).

1. **Diagnosis**

a. Culture and Gram's stain of appropriate specimens.

b. Obtain latex agglutination of CIE tests of urine, tracheal secretions, serum, CSF, to detect group B streptococcus antigen.

2. **Management**

a. Some group B streptococci exhibit tolerance to penicillin-type drugs, and the combination of ampicillin and an aminoglycoside is recommended for a more rapid bactericidal effect.

b. Routine exchange transfusion is of unproven value in group B streptococcus infection, but exchange transfusion with blood containing antibody to the appropriate group B streptococcus serotype improves survival.

c. Antimicrobial treatment of maternal carriers of group B streptococcus has not been shown to prevent group B streptoccocal infection in the neonate.

C. LISTERIOSIS
The etiologic agent is *Listeria monocytogenes.* (A limited number of serotypes account for human infections.)

1. Presentation/Clinical Course

a. Infection in newborns has a biomodal distribution with *early onset* septicemic infection associated with low birth weight, obstetric complications, and maternal colonization. Intrauterine infection may produce a serious granulomatous interstitial pneumonia with high mortality rate. *Late onset* disease tends to occur in infants with normal birth weight with meningitis as a prominent finding and is frequently associated with maternal colonization or obstetric complications.

2. Management

a. Antimicrobic treatment with ampicillin plus gentamicin.

b. Duration of treatment depends on clinical syndrome, e.g., sepsis seven to ten days, meningitis 14 days.

c. Some authorities advocate treatment with penicillin or ampicillin alone.

d. Virtually all listeria exhibit tolerance to penicillin-type drugs, and the addition of an aminoglycoside is recommended for enhanced bactericidal effect.

D. ANAEROBIC INFECTION

Bacteroides fragilis, Peptococcus and *Peptostreptococcus, Veillonella* and *Clostridium perfringens* are most common. Associated with PROM, maternal amnionitis, prematurity, fetal distress; perforated intestine in older neonate, Anaerobes may cause transient bacteremia.

TABLE 10–5.—MANAGEMENT OF INFANT WITH POSSIBLE OR DEFINITE SYPHILIS

STATUS OF INFANT	MATERNAL STATUS	ASSESSMENT	MANAGEMENT
Asymptomatic; positive VDRL; negative FTA-ABS	Asymptomatic; Positive VDRL; Negative FTA-ABS Mother untreated	False-positive finding for syphilis in mother and infant	No treatment necessary
Asymptomatic; positive VDRL; positive FTA-ABS	Asymptomatic; positive VDRL; positive FTA-ABS	Syphilis in mother Syphilis possible in infant	Treat mother. For infant a. Obtain FTA-ABS IGM If positive treat infant if negative, follow infant serologically (Titer should disappear over time) OR b. If FTA-ABS IGM is unavailable: 1. Treat infant; unwise to delay treatment and follow serologically

Asymptomatic positive VDRL; positive FTA-ABS	Asymptomatic; positive VDRL; positive FTA-ABS; mother treated appropriately with penicillin; maternal titer VDRL falling	Adequate treatment of maternal syphilis Adequate treatment of infant by maternal drug therapy	No treatment necessary for mother or infant; follow mother and infant serologically
Asymptomatic positive VDRL; positive FTA-ABS	Asymptomatic; positive VDRL; positive FTA-ABS; mother treated with Erythromycin; maternal titer VDRL falling	Adequate treatment of maternal syphilis May be inadequate	No treatment of mother. May treat infant OR follow serologically.
Symptomatic positive VDRL; positive FTA-ABS	Asymptomatic; Positive VDRL; Positive FTA-ABS; mother untreated	Syphilis in mother Syphilis in infant	Treat mother Treat infant, follow both serologically

Note: RPR or other reagin test may be substituted for VDRL. MHATP may be substituted for FTA-ABS.

TABLE 10–6.—FEATURES OF EARLY AND DELAYED ONSET GBS INFECTION

	EARLY ONSET	LATE ONSET
Time of onset	Birth to 3 days; often occurs within hours of birth	7–10 days to 4 weeks
Clinical manifestations	Fulminating onset: Apnea; tachypnea, respiratory distress, hypoxemia, shock. Meningitis uncommon	More insidious onset of symptoms; mild to moderately severe illness; meningitis frequently present
Delivery and maternal complications	High incidence	Low incidence
Group B serotypes	All 5 serotypes	Type III accounts for 90%
Prognosis	Poor; mortality (50%–75%)	Fair prognosis; mortality of 10% with meningitis
Transmission	Maternal source	Maternal source, nosocomial source, community source

1. Presentation/Clinical Findings

a. Indistinguishable from those of neonatal sepsis.

b. Foul odor of newborn may be clue.

c. Failure to respond to usual antimicrobic agents may also be a clue to anaerobic infection.

2. Diagnosis

a. *Culture* Suitable specimens include blood, pus, and CSF.

b. *Gram's stain* The presence of organisms on Gram's stain and no growth on routine culture supports the *possibility* of anaerobic infection.

3. Management

a. Ampicillin and gentamicin are of limited value in treating anaerobic infection.

b. *Chloramphenicol* is useful for treatment of anaerobic infections, particularly if CNS infection is present.

c. *Clindamycin* may be used for treatment in the neonate, but its failure to diffuse into the CSF makes it inappropriate for treatment of meningitis or brain abscess.

d. *Metronidazole* may be useful in some cases, including CNS infection, but there is limited experience with this drug in infants.

e. *Penicillin* is the drug of choice for clostridia and anaerobic streptococci.

E. TUBERCULOSIS

Neonatal tuberculosis is very rare; a more common problem is the management of an infant of a tuberculous mother, or mother with a positive purified protein derivative (PPD) result. Congenital tuberculosis is a devastating infection usually resulting in abortion or stillbirth. A surviving infant may show nonspecific findings, e.g., low birth weight, poor feeding, listlessness, and hepatomegaly.

1. Diagnosis

a. Acid-fast stain and mycobacterial culture of tracheal aspirates, urine, gastric aspirates, and placenta.

b. Pathologic examination of placenta.

    c. Intermediate (5 T.U.) PPD (often negative).

    d. Review maternal status and results of maternal tests.

2. **Management** Consult Table 10–7.

F. STAPHYLOCOCCUS EPIDERMIDIS

A common saprophyte of skin and mucous membranes, this gram-positive coccus has emerged as a significant pathogen in the neonate, producing pneumonia and sepsis.

1. **Diagnosis** may be suggested by clinical course in association with laboratory findings of thrombocytopenia, metabolic acidosis, glucose intolerance.

    a. Blood culture is definitive procedure.

    b. Endotracheal aspirate culture.

2. **Management**

    a. Removal of contaminated deep line is critical.

    b. Commonly resistant. Use vancomycin until antibiotic susceptibilities are available.

IV. ANTIMICROBIC AGENTS

Special problems related to antimicrobic use in the neonate include differences in volume of distribution of drugs and immaturity of pathways involved in the metabolism and excretion. Dosing is based on serum levels of antimicrobics in infants of similar age, weight, and maturity. If a potentially toxic agent is used, monitor serum levels. Antimicrobics are generally given by the parenteral route (IV or IM) because of the need to ensure adequate serum levels. Intravenous treatment is preferred over IM injections because of the limited muscle mass. Avoid occasional adverse reactions by diluting the drug and running the solution in over 30 minutes rather than giving a bolus push.

A. RECOMMENDED INITIAL DOSES FOR ANTIMICROBICS COMMONLY USED IN THE NEONATE Consult Table 10–8. The following comments apply to dosage recommendations:

1. When treating sepsis of the newborn with penicillin or ampi-

cillin it is recommended that the "meningitis" dose be used as the initial treatment pending results of CSF culture.

2. Chloramphenicol and gentamicin probably should not be used together for treatment since the chloramphenicol antagonizes the antibacterial effect of gentamicin.

B. MONITORING OF ANTIMICROBIC LEVELS

1. **Measure Serum Antimicrobic Levels**   to ensure adequacy of dosage and avoid toxic reaction. Measure CSF bactericidal levels, especially in gram-negative meningitis.

2. **When Microbiologic Assays Are Used for Serum Antimicrobic Determinations**   the laboratory must be aware of *all* antimicrobics the patient is receiving so that an appropriate assay organism is selected or the appropriate chemical means are used to inactivate other antimicrobics in the assay system.

3. **Toxic Levels**   of commonly used drugs are noted in Table 10–9.

4. **Peak Levels**   generally are sampled 30 mintues AFTER the conclusion of a 30-minute IV infusion or one hour after an IM injection.

5. **Trough Levels**   may be measured just before the next dose of antimicrobic.

6.a. The doses of *aminoglycosides* and *chloramphenicol* should be based on serum levels at peak and trough times after the third dose.

   b. Patients with shock or renal compromise should have serum levels monitored after the first dose.

V. NONBACTERIAL NEONATAL INFECTION

A. CYTOMEGALOVIRUS (CMV)

1. **Incidence**   Very common, occurring in 1% to 2% of newborns with higher rates in lower socioeconomic populations.

TABLE 10–7.—MANAGEMENT OF THE TUBERCULOUS OR POTENTIALLY
TUBERCULOUS INFANT

STATUS OF INFANT	MATERNAL STATUS	MANAGEMENT
Symptomatic	Active untreated disease or noncomplaint	1. Treat infant with INH, rifampin 2. Separate infant from mother 3. Review maternal status and assure treatment
Asymptomatic	Active disease; untreated or noncomplaint	1. Isolate infant from mother until latter is noninfectious then: 2. INH prophylaxis 10 mg/kg once daily for infant - apply intermed. (5 T.U.) PPD at 3 months -If negative, discontinue INH, -If positive, reevaluate infant for tuberculosis. If disease is absent continue INH prophylaxis for 1 year; if disease is present, treat for disease with INH plus rifampin OR

		3. High-risk settings BCG infant at birth; return to mother when 5 T.U. PPD is positive (6–8 wk); follow infant
Asymptomatic	On treatment for pulmonary TBC	1. Separate infant from mother until latter is noncontagious
		2. Follow infant; apply 5 T.U. PPD at 3 mo
		-If positive evaluate for tuberculosis and treat accordingly.
		-If negative continue to follow and repeat PPD at 6–9 mo
Asymptomatic	Adequately treated mother OR Mother with positive PPD only	1. Separation of infant from mother unnecessary
		2. Follow infant with 5 T.U. PPD at 3 mo
		3. INH prophylaxis in untreated PPD-positive mother should be considered
		4. Treated mother should be followed to R/O relapse

TABLE 10–8.—DOSES AND SCHEDULES FOR ANTIMICROBICS AGENTS

ANTIMICROBIC AGENT	ROUTE	TOTAL DAILY DOSE (NO. OF DOSES)	
		INFANTS (<1 WK)	INFANTS (1–4 WK)
Ampicillin	IV or IM	50–100 mg/kg (2)	100–150 mg/kg (3)
for meningitis	IV or IM	100–150 mg/kg (2)	200 mg/kg (3)
Carbenicillin	IV or IM	200 mg/kg (2)	300–400 mg/kg (3–4)
Ticarcillin	IV or IM	150 mg/kg (2)	300 mg/kg (3–4)
Mezlocillin	IV or IM	150 mg/kg (2)	300 mg/kg (3–4)
Aqueous penicillin G	IV or IM	100,000 units/kg (2)	100,000 units/kg (3)
for meningitis	IV or IM	150,000 units/kg (2)	200,000 units/kg (3)
Nafcillin	IV or IM	50–100 mg/kg (2)	100–150 mg/kg (3)
Methicillin	IV or IM	50–100 mg/kg (2)	100–200 mg/kg (4)
Gentamicin	IV or IM	5 mg/kg (2)**	7.5 mg/kg (3)**

Drug	Route		
Tobramycin	IV or IM	3.0 mg/kg (1) for infants <2,000 gm** 5 mg/kg (2)**	5.0 mg/kg (2) for infants <2,000 gm** 7.5 mg/kg (3)**
Amikacin	IV or IM	15–20 mg/kg (2)** ?15 mg/kg (1) for infants <2,000 gm**	20–30 mg/kg (2–3) 15–22.5 mg/kg (2) for infants <2,000 gm**
Chloramphenicol	IV	25 mg/kg (1)	25–50 mg/kg (2)
Vancomycin	IV or IM	30 mg/kg (2)	45 mg/kg (3)
Rifampin	Orally	?10 mg/kg (1)	?10–20 mg/kg (1)
Cefazolin	IV or IM	40 mg/kg (2)	40–60 mg/kg (2 or 3)
Moxalactam	IV or IM	100 mg/kg (2)*	150 mg/kg (3)*
Cefotaxime	IV or IM	100 mg/kg (2)	150 mg/kg (3)

*Give loading dose of 100 mg/kg prior to this dosing schedule for gram-negative meningitis.

**Dosage depends on serum concentrations achieved.

Adapted from McCracken G.H., Siegel J.D.: Clinical Pharmacology of Antimicrobial Agents, in Remington J.S., Klein J.O. (eds): *Infectious Disease of the Fetus and Newborn.* Philadelphia, W. B. Saunders Company, 1983, p. 1090.

TABLE 10–9.—"Toxic" Serum Levels for
Various Antimicrobic Agents

ANTIMICROBIC	PEAK	TROUGH
Aminoglycosides		
Gentamicin	>10 μg/ml	>2 μg/ml
Tobramycin	>10 μg/ml	>2 μg/ml
Kanamycin	>40 μg/ml	>10 μg/ml
Amikacin	>40 μg/ml	>10 μg/ml
Chloramphenicol	>25 μg/ml	>10 μg/ml
Penicillin-type drugs*		
Aqueous penicillin G	>200 μg/ml	
Ampicillin	>200 μg/ml	
Carbenicillin	>250 μg/ml	
Nafcillin	>150 μg/ml	
Vancomycin	>40 μg/ml	>5 μg/ml

*There is a great tolerance for high serum levels of these drugs. Only in serious renal failure (for drugs other than nafcillin) or in serious hepatic failure (e.g., nafcillin) is it necessary to reduce dosage.

2. Predisposing Factors/Pathogenesis

a. About 50% of fetuses will become infected during *primary* maternal CMV infection.

b. Infection occurs in about 10% of pregnancies with *recurrent* or reactivated maternal CMV infection.

c. Significant neurological sequelae have been documented following ONLY *primary* maternal infection.

d. CMV infection acquired during the birth process, via breast feeding, or from blood transfusions has not been associated with severe neurological deficits.

e. The probability that a pregnant woman susceptible to CMV will develop a primary infection during a particular pregnancy is less than one in 100. If she does have a primary infection, the changes are one in two that her infant will have congenital infection and one in 14 that will have some residual damage.

3. Presentation/Clinical Course

a. Most infections are clinically inapparent. Late sequelae such as nerve deafness, learning difficulties, and neurological deficits may develop in 10% to 15% of clinically inapparent infections.

b. Syndrome of congenital CMV (cytomegalic inclusion disease [CID]) includes low birth weight, purpura, anemia, jaundice, hepatosplenomegaly, microcephaly, and chorioretinitis. Developmental anomalies are uncommon. The full-blown syndrome is rare.

c. A more common symptomatic presentation is low birth weight, hepatosplenomegaly, and persistent jaundice.

d. Natal/postnatal disease. The incubation period of CMV is probably a minimum of three weeks after which the infant may show signs of hepatosplenomegaly, lymphadenopathy, pneumonia, and atypical lymphocytes. Severe interstitial pneumonia, or transfusion-acquired CMV, may be fatal in premature infants.

4. Diagnosis

a. Infants with congenital infection excrete CMV in high titer in urine and saliva, making virus detection easy and rapid.
  i. Collect saliva specimens in viral culture medium and keep on ice. Urine specimens should be sent on ice to laboratory.
  ii. Do not freeze specimens. (Freezing inactivates the virus).

b. Specific CMV IgM may be detected in cord or infant serum.

c. Electron microscopy studies of saliva, urinary sediment, or liver tissue may demonstrate CMV viral particles.

d. Look for typical large cells with inclusions by cytologic examination of urinary sediment or in liver tissue.

e. IgG CMV antibody in persistent high titer at 6 to 12 weeks of age supports diagnosis.

f. Additional diagnostic studies to determine extent of infection include skull film or CT scan for detection of intracranial calcifications, liver function tests, long-bone films, and chest x-ray films.

5. Management

a. No specific, effective antiviral therapy exists.

b. Newborn hearing screening is important, e.g., brain-stem auditory evoked response. Repeated evaluations are indicated since postnatal development of deafness occurs.

c. Infants with congenital CMV infection may infect otners.

Some authorities suggest susceptible pregnant nurses should not care for these infants.

d. Prevention of neonatal CMV infection via blood transfusion in susceptible premature infants may be accomplished by use of CMV antibody–negative blood for transfusion.

e. Prevention of symptomatic congenital CMV infection is not possible. A live virus vaccine is under investigation.

REFERENCES

1. Stagno S., Pass R.F., Dworsky M.E., et al.: Congenital cytomegalovirus infection. The relative importance of primary and recurrent maternal infection. *N. Engl. J. Med.* 306:945–949, 1982.
2. Kumar M.L., Nankervis G.A., Gold E.: Inapparent CMV infection: A follow-up study. *N. Engl. J. Med.* 288:1370–1372, 1973.
3. Yeager A.S., Grumet F.C., Hafleigh E.B., et al.: Prevention of transfusion-acquired cytomegalovirus infections in newborn infants. *J. Pediatr.* 98:281–287, 1981.
4. Ballard R.A., Drew W.L., Hufnagle K.G., et al.: Acquired cytomegalovirus infection in preterm infants. *AJDC* 133:482–485, 1979.

B. RUBELLA

Only 19 cases of congenital rubella syndrome (CRS) were reported in 1981, reflecting the success of rubella vaccine. All personnel in contact with CRS should have antibody to rubella either as a result of prior infection or immunization.

1. Signs and Symptoms

Developmental anomalies occur primarily as a result of infection in the first trimester and involve the heart (patent ductus arteriosis [PDA], peripheral pulmonic stenosis, ventricular septal defect [VSD], atrial septal defect), eye (glaucoma, cataracts, chorioretinitis), and ear (nerve deafness).

a. Vaccination should not be given during pregnancy, but inadvertent administration carries a very low risk of fetal disease.

b. Sequelae of persistent viral infection are growth retardation, abnormal liver function, anemia, thrombocytopenia, CNS damage, immune deficiencies, and dental dysplasia.

c. Considerable overlap exists in clinical manifestations of CMV, herpes, toxoplasmosis, syphilis, and rubella. Heart lesions are more likely in rubella.

2. Diagnosis

a. Isolation of virus from urine and throat (infants with CRS may excrete virus months to years).

b. Specific rubella IgM antibody or persistence of rubella IgG antibody in infant.

3. Management/Prevention

a. There is no specific antiviral chemotherapy.

b. Appropriate treatment of specific defects should be given.

c. Respiratory and enteric isolation of infants with CRS is required.

C. HERPES SIMPLEX VIRUS (HSV)

Two serotypes are recognized: HSV 1 and HSV 2. Either type causes severe disease with high mortality and morbidity in the neonate.

1. **Incidence** Estimates vary from 1:7,500 to 1:30,000 pregnancies, or about 120 cases of neonatal HSV infection in the United States each year.

2. **Predisposing Factors/Pathogenesis** Transplacental infection resulting in abortion or congenital malformations occurs rarely. The most common route of infection is via contact with maternal genital secretions. Inoculation of the virus occurs at skin trauma sites, e.g., fetal scalp monitors; nosocomial spread is possible.

3. **Signs and Symptoms** vary with the type of disease. Asymptomatic infection is rare. Localized skin or eye involvement occurs. Disseminated disease may present with findings described for sepsis; localized CNS disease may present with fever, lethargy, poor feeding hypoglycemia, disseminated intravascular coagulation (DIC), and irritability followed by intractable focal or generalized seizures. Vesicular lesions, when present, are an important clue to diagnosis.

4. **Diagnostic Efforts**

a. Scrape the base of vesicles and lesions for Tzanck smear to demonstrate multinucleated giant cells characteristic of herpes viruses or for direct immunofluorescent test for herpes simplex antigen.

b. Obtain a viral culture from vesicles, blood, throat, CSF, or eye lesions. Brain biopsy may be done in the appropriate setting.

c. Examine the mother for vaginal, cervical, or other herpes lesions, but culture for virus even in the absence of lesions.

d. Tests for herpes simplex antibody in mother and infant have not proved helpful diagnostically.

5. Management

a. Antiviral drug therapy is indicated for all forms of neonatal herpes infection since even initially localized disease may disseminate with devastating effects. Currently available treatment consists of adenine arabinoside, 30 mg/kg/day given as a 12-hour IV infusion for ten days.

b. Infant must be isolated.

c. Acyclovir, another antiviral agent, is being evaluated for efficacy in drug therapy of neonatal herpes infection. It may prove more effective than ARA.

REFERENCES

1. Whitley R.J., Nahmias A.J., Visintine A.M., et al.: The natural history of herpes simplex virus infection of mother and newborn. *Pediatrics* 66:489, 1980.
2. Arvin A.M., Yeager A.S., Bruhn F.W., et al.: Neonatal herpes simplex infection in the absence of mucocutaneous lesions. J. Pediatr. 100:715–721, 1982.

D. HEPATITIS

Neonatal hepatitis may have multiple infectious causes (Table 10–10). Hepatitis A (HAV) and B (HBV) will be discussed in this section.

1. Hepatitis A (HAV)

a. *Incidence* Unknown. Transmission of HAV to the neonate is possible if the mother is in the incubation period or is acutely symptomatic at the time of delivery. In infected children the virus is detectable in the stool for two weeks before onset of clinical illness and for several days afterward.

b. *Diagnosis* HAV infection is established by detecting antigen in the stool (not routinely available) or by finding anti-HAV-IGM antibody in serum specimens.

ZZMISC

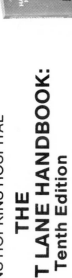

TABLE 10–10.—CAUSES OF INFECTIOUS
NEONATAL HEPATITIS

VIRAL*	OTHER
Hepatitis A, B, non-A, non-B	Bacterial sepsis
Rubella	Syphilis
CMV	Listeria
Herpes simplex	Tuberculosis
Enteroviruses	Toxoplasmosis
Coxsackie	
ECHO	
Adenovirus	
Varicella	

*CMV indicates cytomegalovirus; ECHO, echoviruses.

c. *Management*
   i. Enteric precautions are recommended for one week after onset of jaundice or abnormal liver function test results.
  ii. In the infant born to an acutely symptomatic mother, ISG .02 ml/kg IM should be considered although its effectiveness is unknown. The occurrence of HAV infection earlier in pregnancy is not an indication for withholding breast-feeding or administration of immune serum globulin.

2. Hepatitis B (HBV)

a. *Incidence* Varies with ethnic origin of mother, the timing and type of maternal infection, whether or not mother is HBsAg and "e" positive.

b. *Predisposing factors/pathogenesis*
   i. Transplacental transmission is rare. Transmission to an infant by HBsAg-positive mothers occurs during or shortly after delivery (Table 10–11). HBIG and Hepatavax are used to protect the infant from acute infection and development of chronic infection.
  ii. A mother with acute (symptomatic) hepatitis late in pregnancy or shortly after delivery is much *more* likely to transmit infection to her infant than a mother with acute infection early in pregnancy or the mother who is a chronic carrier.
  iii. *But* the infected infant of a chronic carrier is most likely to develop severe chronic liver disease.
  iv. Chronic severe liver disease is more common in Asians.

TABLE 10–11.—WOMEN AT HIGHER RISK OF BEING HBsAg POSITIVE

1. Women with acute or chronic liver disease
2. Women of Asian, Pacific Islander, native Alaskan descent, or from Haiti or subsaharan Africa
3. Women rejected as blood donors
4. Women who work or receive treatment in a renal dialysis unit (including spouses)
5. Women who work or reside as patients in an institution for the retarded
6. Women who have illicitly used drugs by the percutaneous route
7. Women who live with persons acutely or chronically infected with hepatitis B virus (HBsAg carriers)
8. Women with medical problems who have received repeated blood transfusions
9. Women who have frequent occupational exposure to blood in medical-dental settings

   c. *Presentation/clinical course*
      i. Most infants who develop HBV infection, i.e., become HBsAg positive as a result of maternal transmission, remain clinically well. Persistent antigenemia may develop (Table 10–12).
      ii. Some infants (1% to 3%) may become icteric, have elevated liver enzyme levels, and otherwise do poorly; these are most likely to be the offspring of "e" positive carrier mothers.
      iii. Fulminant hepatitis in the newborn is rare.

TABLE 10–12.—RISK OF HBV TRANSMISSION FROM MOTHER TO INFANT AND OUTCOME FOR INFANT

MOTHER HBsAg POSITIVE	INFECTION RATE FOR INFANT, %	CHRONIC CARRIER RISK IN INFANT, %
Acute hepatitis 3 mo before to 1 mo after delivery	80–90	
Acute hepatitis in early pregnancy	10–30	
Asymptomatic carrier mother	10	
HBeAg positive	90	85–90
HBeAg negative	30	Low
HBeAg negative, anti–BHe positive	Very low	Very low

   iv. HBsAg carriers have increased risk for later development of hepatocellular carcinoma (HCC). Lack of precise knowledge concerning the long-term effect of HBV in the newborn makes it prudent to prevent infection whenever possible.

d. *Diagnosis* Detection of specific antigens and antibodies is the means by which HBV infection is established.
   i. HBsAg positivity indicates either acute HBV infection or the presence of carrier state.
   ii. HBeAg positivity, detectable only in the presence of HBsAg, indicates infectiveness and increased likelihood of transmission of HBV.
   iii. Anti-HBs in serum indicates past infection with HBV and immunity to HBV.
   iv. Anti-HBc in serum indicates recent, chronic, or remote HBV infection.

e. *Management*
   i. Screen mothers in high-risk groups for HBsAg (see Table 10–11).
   ii. Newborns of HBsAg-positive mothers or high-risk mothers of unknown HBsAg status should receive 0.5 cc IM of HBIG *in the delivery room.*
   iii. HB vaccine (0.5 cc IM) should be administered within 7 days, at 1 month, and at 6 months if mother is HBsAg-positive.
   iv. Infants with documented HBV infection should be isolated; blood and secretion precautions are indicated.
   v. After thorough bathing and rinsing, isolation of a newborn born to a carrier is not necessary.
   vi. Strict isolation or separation of the carrier mother and/or her infant is *not* indicated. Breast-feeding is permitted.
   vii. Infants treated with HBIG and vaccine should be followed up at 12 to 15 months of age to determine the success of treatment.
   viii. The use of HBIG and vaccine can prevent approximately 90% of neonatal and subsequent HBV infections.

REFERENCES

1. Beasely R.P., Hwang L.Y., Lin C.C., et al.: Hepatitis B immune globulin (HBIG) efficacy in the interruption of perinatal transmission of hepatitis B virus carrier state. *Lancet* 2:388–393, 1981.
2. Szmuness W., Stevens C.E., Zang E.A., et al.: A controlled clinical trail of the efficacy of the hepatitis B vaccine (Heptavax B). *Hepatology* 1:377–385, 1982.
3. Past exposure prophylaxis hepatitis B. *MMWR* 33:285, 1984.

E. ENTEROVIRUSES

Polio, Coxsackie virus, and echoviruses constitute this group.

1. **Incidence** Undetermined; seasonal occurrence in summer and fall, more common in males.

2. **Predisposing Factors/Pathogenesis**

   a. Infection may be acquired congenitally, natally, or postnatally. Onset of symptoms at birth suggests late-gestation congenital infection, onset of disease at five to ten days suggests acquisition natally, and onset of disease beyond ten days suggests postnatal acquisition.

   b. Coxsackie infection during pregnancy may be associated with congenital malformation of cardiovascular, urogenital, and digestive systems in the neonate. Coxsackie B infections are more virulent than echoviruses or Coxsackie A.

3. **Presentation/Clinical Course**

   a. Fever and other nonspecific signs and symptoms as in sepsis are usual. Maculopapular or petechial rash may occur. Occasionally infections are asymptomatic.

   b. More virulent infection is seen with meningitis, encephalitis, or myocarditis. Fulminant illness with jaundice, pulmonary infiltrates, diarrhea, DIC, and necrosis of adrenals and pancreas is less common.

4. **Diagnosis**

   a. Recovery of enterovirus from CSF, biopsy, or autopsy tissue.

   b. Recovery of enterovirus from stool or pharyngeal secretions is suggestive of causal relationship to illness.

   c. A documented rise in antibody titer to viral isolate supports the diagnosis.

5. **Management**

   a. No specific antiviral drug treatment.

   b. Supportive care for myocardial, hepatic, and CNS involvement.

   c. Vigorous infection control measures are indicated, including enteric isolation precautions, emphasis on hand-washing among personnel, and exclusion of personnel with symptoms of enteroviral disease from nursery.

REFERENCES

1. Wilfert C.M., Thompson R.J. Jr., Sunder T.R., et al.: Longitudinal assessment of children with enteroviral meningitis during the first three months of life. *Pediatrics* 67:811–815, 1981.
2. Kibrick S.: Viral infection of the fetus and newborn. *Perspect. Virol.* 2:140–159, 1961.
3. Modlin J.F., Polk B.F., Horton P., et al.: Perinatal echovirus infection: Risk of transmission during a community outbreak. *N. Engl. J. Med.* 305:368–371, 1981.

F. VARICELLA ZOSTER (VZ)

1. **Incidence**   Ninety percent of women in the childbearing age are immune. Congenital and neonatal varicella are rare (Table 10–13).

2. **Presentation/Clinical Course**

   a. Congenital defects due to maternal VZ infection in the first and second trimester have been associated with cutaneous scars, abnormalities of digits or a limb, defects of eye, brain, and low birth weight in newborns.

   b. Newborns acquiring VZ infection during the perinatal period have a clinical illness varying from mild to fatal. The acquisition of transplacental antibody determines the outcome in infants.

3. **Diagnosis**

   a. *Congenital varicella*   Specific IgM VZ antibody or persistence of significant titers of VZ IgG.

   b. *Neonatal varicella*
      i. Characteristic diffusely disseminated skin lesions in varying stages, from macules, papules, vesicles, pustules, and crusts, are present.
      ii. Recovery of VZ virus by culture.
      iii. Immunofluorescent staining of scrapings.
      iv. Tzanck smear of vesicle base scrapings will show multinucleated giant cells in both VZ and herpes simplex infections.

4. **Management**

   a. Infants with *congenital* varicella do not require isolation.

   b. Infants with *neonatal* varicella should be placed in strict isolation for at least seven days after onset of rash.

TABLE 10–13.—Neonatal Chickenpox Secondary to Maternal Varicella

DISEASE ONSET IN MOTHER	DISEASE ONSET IN INFANT	NO. OF INFANTS	FATALITY, NO. (%)
5 or more days before delivery	0–4 days of age	27	0 (0)
0–4 days before delivery	5–10 days of age	23	7 (30)

c. The use of adenine arabinoside has not been evaluated. Infants born to mothers with onset of varicella five or more days before to delivery require no specific treatment other than isolation if kept in hospital.

d. Infants whose mothers have onset of varicella from zero to four days before delivery, or within two days after delivery, should receive one vial (2.5 ml) of VZIG, preferably at birth or within 96 hours.

e. Infants who may be exposed to VZ infection as a result of contact with nursery personnel should have their immune status verified and if susceptible should receive VZIG, 2.5 ml, within 96 hours of exposure. Premature infants are more susceptible.

REFERENCES

1. Gershon A.A.: Varicella in mother and infant, in Krugman S., Gershon A.A. (eds.): *Infections of the Fetus and Newborn Infant.* New York, A.R. Liss, 1975.

G. CANDIDA ALBICANS

1. Predisposing Factors/Pathogenesis

a. *Rarely*—Candida infection may occur in utero by blood stream invasion or more likely as the result of ascending infection.

b. *Very commonly*—Neonatal infection results from contamination during the birth process or nosocomial transmission.

c. Dissemination of candidal infection may occur postnatally in association with antibiotic usage, indwelling catheters, TPN, steroids, and in otherwise stressed neonates.

2. Presentation/Clinical Course

a. Superficial infection is common. Creamy white patches adherent to mucous membranes (thrush) or in the diaper area, well-defined satelliting erythematous vesiculo-pustules associated with confluent erythematous macules may be found.

b. Congenital *disseminated* candidiasis may involve kidney, lungs, liver, brain, eye, and organs, or present as a localized infection, e.g., candidal arthritis or candidal meningitis. A generalized maculopapular-vesicular rash may be present. Course without treatment is ordinarily fatal.

c. Congenital cutaneous candidiasis is superficial and confined to skin and umbilical cord. It may occur with intact membranes. Manifestations include a diffuse maculopapular-vesicular rash distributed over the face, trunk, neck, and limbs. Desquamation follows the acute phase. No constitutional symptoms are present and the infant thrives. Cutaneous candidiasis must be distinguished from erythema toxicum, congenital herpes, syphilis, or bullous impetigo.

3. Diagnosis

a. Isolation on ordinary blood agar as well as fungal culture medium should be done. Recovery from blood culture may represent a transient candidemia or disseminated infection.

b. Gram's stain may yield large, gram-positive, watermelon-seed–shaped yeast cells. At times hyphae with budding yeast cells are seen.

c. Tissue diagnosis from biopsy specimens should be done.

e. Ophthalmologic examination is indicated in suspected disseminated candidiasis.

4. Management

a. Treatment of localized oral or GI tract candidiasis is nystatin, 200,000 units orally four times daily for one week or longer.

b. Skin lesions may be treated with topical nystatin or amphotericin B ointment applied four times daily for a week.

c. Disseminated candidiasis requires treatment with amphotericin B and flucytosine pending determination of fungal sensitivity studies.

REFERENCES

1. Keller M.A., Sellers B.B.J., Melish M.E., et al.: Systemic candidiasis in infants. *AJDC* 131:1260–1263, 1977.
2. Johnson D.E., Thompson T.R., Ferrieri P.: Congenital candidiasis. *AJDC* 135:273–275, 1981.

H. TOXOPLASMOSIS

An infection caused by a common obligate intracellular parasite of birds and mammals, *Toxoplasma gondii*. Cats are the definitive host.

1. Incidence
Approximately 3,300 cases of congenital infection occur yearly in the United States.

2. Predisposing Factors/Pathogenesis

a. Only *primary* infection of the mother, which is usually asymptomatic, results in congenital infection. Ninety percent of offspring of women who acquired infection during pregnancy appear normal, and 50% of these escape infection. Of the remaining 10%, most have minor problems and only 3% to 5% have severe manifestations. Overall, 75% of congenitally infected infants are asymptomatic.

b. Transplacental transmission of maternal parasitemia increases from about 15% in the first trimester to about 65% at the end of the pregnancy.

3. Presentation/Clinical Course

a. The classic triad of hydrocephalus, chorioretinitis, and intracranial calcification occurs in infants infected early in pregnancy.
   i. These infants may also appear septic and have jaundice, hepatosplenomegaly, purpura, deafness, chorioretinitis.
   ii. Differentiation from other congenital infections, e.g., herpes simplex, CMV, rubella, or syphilis, requires laboratory support.

b. Infants infected late in pregnancy usually appear clinically normal.

4. Diagnosis   A variety of serological procedures are available for diagnosis:

a. *Sabin dye test*   Sensitive and very specific, but requirement for live parasites in test makes it unavailable in most diagnostic laboratories.

b. *Indirect fluorescent antibody test (IFA)*   More readily available and most routinely used test.

c. *IgM-IFA*   Detects early antibody in acute infection, but not routinely available. Theoretically the test of choice for congenital toxoplasmosis. However, there are technical problems with the test. Also, some congenitally infected infants lack IgM-IFA antibody.

d. A rising dye or IFA titer, the disappearance of IgM-IFA titer, or both of these occurring over an interval of several weeks generally establishes the diagnosis. A single high titer, while suspicious, *does not* establish the diagnosis.

e. Recovery of parasites from infected tissues, bone marrow, or blood is possible in tissue culture or after inoculation in mice (not routinely available).

5. Management

a. Fully satisfactory therapy for toxoplasmosis is not available.

b. Pyrimethamine/sulfadiazine combination
   i. Sulfadiazine, 150 mg/kg/day in four doses for one month—not to exceed 4 g daily.
   ii. Pyrimethamine, 1 mg/kg/day in two doses for one month—not to exceed 25 mg total daily dose.
   iii. (A loading dose of pyrimethamine of 2 mg/kg/day in two doses for two to three days is given. This dose may exceed 25 mg/day).
   iv. Folinic acid, 5 to 10 mg/kg/day should also be administered to prevent hematologic toxic reaction.

c. Congenitally infected newborns should probably be treated to prevent progression of disease. In asymptomatic infants the prevention of development of debilitating consequences is the aim of treatment. In face of a high stable titer of IgG antibody without clinical illness in early infancy, one may either treat or follow the patient carefully monthly with toxititers and for evidence of disease (eye findings, failure to thrive).

REFERENCES

1. Remington J.S., Desmonds G.: Toxoplasmosis, In Remington J.S., Klein J.O. (eds.): *Infectious Disease of the Fetus and Newborn Infant.* Philadelphia, W.B. Saunders Co., 1983.
2. Wilson C.B., Remington J.S., Stagno S., et al.: Development of adverse sequellae in children with subclinical congenital Toxoplasma infection. *Pediatrics* 66:767–774, 1980.

11

Intraventricular Hemorrhage (IVH)

A. INCIDENCE

1. IVH occurs in about 40% of premature infants weighing less than 1,500 gm.

2. About 8% of infants under 1,500 gm have intraparenchymal hemorrhage as well.

B. CLASSIFICATION

1. Ultrasound/CT scan classification

a. Grade I—subependymal hemorrhage.

b. Grade II—IVH without ventricular dilatation.

c. Grade III—IVH with ventricular dilatation.

d. Grade IV—intraventricular and intraparenchymal hemorrhage.

2. Neuropathological classification

a. *Primary lesion* Bleeding from small vessels in the highly vascularized subependymal germinal matrix, most often overlying the head of the caudate nucleus.

b. *Intraventricular extension* Rupture of the matrix hemorrhage through the ependyma.

c. *Intraparenchymal hemorrhage* Probably represents ischemic infarction rather than "extension" of IVH, and usually involves destruction of brain beyond the borders of hemorrhage.

d. *Hydrocephalus*
   i. Acute hydrocephalus may occur with large IVH, probably

as a result of acute obstruction of extraventricular flow by blood clot.

ii. Delayed or slowly progressive hydrocephalus probably results from an obliterative arachnoiditis.

C. PATHOGENESIS

Factors thought to predispose premature infants to IVH include the following:

1. Immaturity of the subependymal germinal matrix and vascular bed.

   a. Gelatinous area with poor support of rich vascular network.

   b. Capillary endothelium probably has high dependency on oxidative metabolism and is vulnerable to hypoxic damage.

   c. Periventricular region contains a large amount of fibrinolytic activity.

2. Poor autoregulation of cerebral blood flow in the periventricular region.

   a. Blood flow is pressure dependent, resulting in large fluctuations with variation in BP.

   b. Intracapillary pressure may be sensitive to acute elevations in venous pressure, e.g., with pneumothorax, exchange transfusion.

3. Minor defects in hemostatic mechanisms, e.g., fibrinogen, may play a role in hemorrhages that progress over time.

D. DIAGNOSIS

1. Symptoms include shock, acidosis, anemia, pallor, change in neurological status, seizures, acute change in lung compliance and requirements for ventilatory assistance, apnea, and bradycardia. Most hemorrhages are asymptomatic.

2. Onset of IVH

   a. About 50% will occur within the first day of life.

   b. About 85% will occur within the first three days of life.

3. Portable real-time ultrasonography is the method of choice. Computed tomographic scanning requires transporting the patient and generally is not required.

4. We recommend that all premature infants under 1,500 gm have a diagnostic ultrasound in the first week of life.

E. PREVENTION AND TREATMENT

1. Proposed methods to prevent IVH are unproven or controversial.

   a. Sedation with phenobarbital to prevent fluctuations in BP.

   b. Monitoring venous pressure to maintain stable low venous pressure.

   c. Correction of clotting deficiencies with fresh-frozen plasma.

2. **Acute Management**   Maintain adequate cerebral perfusion.

   a. Maintain normal BP by volume replacement, inotropic agents.

   b. Control cerebral vascular resistance in acute hydrocephalus by lumbar puncture or ventriculostomy.

3. **Posthemorrhagic hydrocephalus**

   a. Follow with serial ultrasound evaluation. Ventriculomegaly will occur before there is an increase in head circumference.

   b. Rapidly expanding hydrocephalus should be treated with repeated ventricular taps until the CSF protein is low or until the infant is large enough to receive a ventriculoperitoneal shunt.

   c. Slowly developing ventricular dilatation may resolve spontaneously or may respond to the following:
      i. Daily lumbar puncture with removal of CSF until flow stops.
      ii. Drugs that decrease CSF formation, e.g., furosemide, acetazolamide.

F. OUTCOME

1. Outcome probably relates to the severity of the hemorrhage and the success in stabilizing the infant's condition and maintaining cerebral perfusion following IVH.

2. A small subependymal hemorrhage or small IVH seems to result in no long-term morbidity.

3. Hydrocephalus per se, if appropriately treated, probably contributes little to subsequent morbidity.

4. In severe IVH, the mortality rate is about 50%, and about 50% of survivors develop hydrocephalus. (Experience varies with institution.)

5. Moderate-to-severe neurological deficits are largely confined to infants with intraparenchymal involvement and its attendant ischemic cerebral damage.

12

Neonatal Seizures

Neonatal seizures occur in one to 15 out of 1,000 live births. Approximately 15% of premature infants in the neonatal intensive care unit setting will have at least one seizure episode. Seizures are an important prognostic indicator for later neurological development.

A. SIGNS AND SYMPTOMS

1. **Subtle, Repetitive "Normal" Activities** These occur in 50% of all seizures.

   a. Sucking, chewing, fluttering eyelids, rowing, pedaling.

   b. Generalized fragmentary seizures—these migrate rapidly and randomly.

2. **Tonic Seizures**

   a. Rigidity, posturing, tonic eye deviation, apnea.

   b. Common in structural brain abnormalities.

   c. Poor prognosis.

3. **Multifocal Clonic**

   a. Can be generalized or local and progressive.

   b. Poor prognosis.

4. **Focal Clonic**

   a. More common after gestational age of 34 weeks.

   b. Good prognosis, with short, intermittent episodes.

5. **Myoclonic Seizures**

   a. Continuous myoclonic episodes, not merely muscle "jerks."

   b. Poor prognosis.

B. DIFFERENTIAL DIAGNOSIS

1. **Apnea**   Usually a secondary symptom.

   a. Occurs without seizures in 25% of premature infants.

   b. The heart rate usually remains unchanged in convulsive apnea.

2. **Jitteriness**   Rhythmic movements that can be altered or eliminated by change in position, or passive flexion of involved extremity.

3. **Rapid Eye Movement (REM) Sleep**   First stage of sleep of infant. Movements are continuous and can be abolished by waking.

4. **Opsoclonus**

   a. Rhythmic, rapid deviation of the eyes.

   b. Associated with structural abnormalities, severe injury, or infection.

C. CAUSES

1. **Hypoxia**—most common.

   a. Asphyxia neonatorum.

   b. Aspiration syndromes.

2. **Intracranial Trauma**

   a. Hemorrhage/hematoma.

   b. Cystic necrosis from prenatal insult.

3. **Metabolic**

   a. Electrolyte abnormality—sodium, calcium, magnesium.

   b. Hypoglycemia.

   c. Pyridoxine deficiency or dependency.

   d. Aminoacidopathies.

   e. Urea cycle abnormalities.

4. **Infection**

   a. *Bacterial—Escherichia coli,* group B *streptococcus, Listeria,* later *S. aureus, S. epidermidis.*

  b. *Viral*—Congenital and acquired.

5. **Maternal Drug Addiction and Subsequent Withdrawal in the Infant**   Opiates, barbiturates, propoxyphene.

6. **Toxic Agents**

  a. Isoniazide

  b. Bilirubin

  c. Local anesthetic agents

7. **Genetic/Dysmorphic Factors**

  a. Chromosomal abnormalities

  b. Phakomatosis, e.g., tuberous sclerosis, neurofibromatosis

  c. Cerebral dysgenesis

  d. Syndrome with mental retardation

  e. Familial epilepsy—uncommon presentation in neonatal period

D. EVALUATION

1. Careful prenatal/perinatal and family history.

2. Thorough physical examination including serial occipital-frontal circumferences (OFCs) and basic reflexes.

3. Serum measurements of glucose, sodium, calcium, magnesium, bicarbonate, BUN, creatinine, bilirubin, and ammonia levels.

4. Arterial blood gas volume.

5. Lumbar puncture to analyze CSF for protein, glucose, blood, WBCs, electrolytes, and bacterial/viral culture.

6. Urine/serum metabolic screen or amino acids.

7. TORCH titers—maternal and infant.

8. CT scan, ultrasound, or both.

  a. Skull x-ray films are of little value in the newborn in differentiating calcifications or location of hemorrhage.

b. Angiogram may occasionally be required for complete evaluation of hemorrhage, infarction, or vascular malformation site.

9. Electroencephalogram (EEG)—maturation occurs at 24 to 40 weeks of gestational age; an EEG is most valuable within the first days of life.

a. EEG findings associated with seizure activity
   i. Migratory sharp waves
   ii. Monorhythmic delta waves
   iii. Spike and wave uncommon in neonate
   iv. Positive and negative spikes at 2 to 6 Hz

b. EEG findings associated with a poor prognosis
   i. Low voltage
   ii. Disorganized activity
   iii. Burst suppression activity in the absence of medication
   iv. Runs of alpha waves.

E. TREATMENT

1. Correct Primary Cause if Possible

a. Avoid cerebral edema
   i. Restrict fluids.
   ii. Mechanical hyperventilation to maintain P_{CO_2} at 20 to 25 torr.

b. Correct metabolic imbalances.
   i. Glucose, 2 to 4 ml/kg D_{25} W IV.
   ii. Calcium, 2 ml/kg of 10% calcium gluconate IV.
   iii. Magnesium, O.2 ml/kg of 50% $MgSO_4$ IM.
   iv. Pyridoxine, 50 to 100 mg of pyridoxine hydrochloride IV for unexplained seizures. In patients with pyridoxine dependency the EEG may sometimes revert to normal immediately, but may take several days to improve.
   v. For metabolic acidosis, give $NaHCO_3$ calculated to provide one half correction. If serum sodium level is high, correct slowly with IV glucose fluids or Tris-hydroxymethyl aminomethane (THAM).

c. Remove toxins if identified.
   i. Peritoneal dialysis, e.g., transient hyperammonemia.
   ii. Exchange transfusion, e.g., kernicterus, hyperammonemia.

d. Use antibiotic therapy for CSF infection if bacterial infection.

2. Anticonvulsant Therapy

a. *Phenobarbital* Long half life.
   i. Loading dose, 20 mg/kg IV.
   ii. Maintenance, 3 to 4 mg/kg/day IV or orally.
   iii. Therapeutic range, 15 to 40 mg/l.

b. *Phenytoin* (Diphenylhydantoin, Dilantin)   Additive effects with phenobarbital.
   i. Loading dose, 20 mg/kg IV. Infuse without dilution at a rate lower than 0.5 mg/kg/min and flush catheter with normal saline immediately (incompatible with glucose solution).
   ii. Maintenance dose, 5 to 8 mg/kg/day IV twice daily.
   iii. Oral and IM administered drug is poorly absorbed in the neonate.
   iv. Therapeutic range, 10 to 20 mg/l.

c. *Primidone* may impair phenobarbital clearance; the neonate apparently does not have the ability to convert primidone to phenobarbital. Primidone is rarely indicated.
   i. Loading dose, 20 mg/kg orally.
   ii. Maintenance dose, 15 mg/kg orally.
   iii. Therapeutic range, 7 to 15 mg/l.

d. *Paraldehyde* Side effects include pulmonary edema/hemorrhage and hypotension in older children; used mainly for status epilepticus. Dose, 0.2 mg/kg IV is recommended.

e. *Diazepam (Valium)* is seldom effective as an additional drug in neonates, and its preservative (sodium benzoate) may displace bilirubin from albumin. For use in uncontrolled status epilepticus, 0.2–0.5 mg/kg/dose IV is recommended.

f. *Barbiturate coma*
   i. Indicated only in severe hypoxic/ischemic brain injury. Benefit in acute neonatal asphyxia is doubtful.
   ii. Possibly acts by increasing free radical scavengers in CNS tissue, blockage metabolic requirements, or calcium channel.
   iii. Side effects include hypotension, cardiovascular collapse, and apnea.
   iv. Method:
   Pentobarbitol, 15–20 mg/kg IV adjusted to keep level at 20 to 40 mg/L.
   Phenobarbitol, 20 to 30 mg/kg IV for the initial dose, then 2 to 5 mg/kg every six hours to maintain level at 60 to 70 mg/l.

TABLE 12-1.—CAUSES AND PROGNOSES OF NEONATAL SEIZURES*

CAUSE OF SEIZURE (NO.)	DIED, %	SURVIVORS			
		NORMAL, %	TOTAL ABNORMAL, %	MINIMAL ABNORMALITY, %	SIGNIFICANT ABNORMALITY, %
Total group	25	62	38	6	32
Hypoxia/trauma (180)	25	53	47	8	39
Unknown cause (139)	9	69	31	6	25
Hypocalcemia (113)	0	95	5	3	2
Infection (52)	35	47	53	...	...
Subarachnoid hemorrhage	11	100	...	...	...
Hypoglycemia (31)	3	50	50	...	...
Malformation (24)	71	0	100	...	...

*Adapted from a literature review by Bergman et al.[1]
Under the best prediction of outcome, the infant appears definitely normal at discharge. The seizure recurrence rate is about 15% overall, and 22% in cases of postseizure hypoxia/trauma.

F. PROGNOSIS

1. **Morbidity + Mortality = 50% Overall.** Death or risk of neurological sequelae depend on etiology (Table 12–1).

   a. Hypoglycemia—50%.

   b. Hypoxia—60%.

   c. Infection—70%.

2. The outlook is good (70% to 80% are normal) if the following occurs:

   a. There are less than four seizures, all of less than ten minutes' duration.

   b. There are less than two days of seizure activity.

   c. The five-minute Apgar is greater than 7.

   d. No resuscitation is required after five-minute Apgar.

REFERENCES

1. Bergman I., Painter M., Crumrine P.K.: Neonatal seizures. *Sem. Perinatol* 6:54–67, 1982.
2. Volpe, J.J.: Management of neonatal seizures. *Crit. Care Med.* 5:43–49, 1977.

13

Pulmonary Diseases

I. RESPIRATORY DISTRESS SYNDROME OR HYALINE MEMBRANE DISEASE

Respiratory distress syndrome is the most common cause of respiratory failure in newborns. It occurs in infants with immature lungs who produce or release inadequate amounts of pulmonary surfactant. Diffuse atelectasis and reduced lung compliance are the major pathophysiological features. The incidence of RDS increases with decreasing gestational age. Infants who are asphyxiated, hypovolemic, or born of diabetic mothers are at increased risk. Infants with congenital pneumonia may have findings that are indistinguishable from RDS.

A. DIAGNOSIS

1. **Clinical Findings** in addition to prematurity include the following:

a. Signs of respiratory distress (tachypnea, chest wall retractions, poor air entry into the lungs by auscultation, nasal flaring, expiratory grunting, and cyanosis).

b. Progressive pulmonary insufficiency (blood gas analysis).

c. Other findings include systemic hypotension, oliguria, hypotonia, temperature instability, and ileus and peripheral edema.

2. **Chest X-ray Film** demonstrates a characteristic reticulogranular or ground-glass pattern and air bronchograms indicating diffuse atelectasis.

3. **Biochemical Findings** include the following:

a. Amniotic fluid L/S ratio less than 2.0, a negative (immature) Shake test finding using gastric aspirate or amniotic fluid, or both.

b. Absence of phosphatidylglycerol from the amniotic fluid.

B. NATURAL HISTORY

1. **Pulmonary Insufficiency** worsens during the first 24 to 48 hours and then plateaus.

2. **Resolution** is frequently preceded by increased urine output usually beginning between 60 and 90 hours of age.

C. MANAGEMENT—GENERAL PRINCIPLES

The object of therapy in RDS is to support the infant until spontaneous resolution occurs. Oxygen consumption and CO_2 production may be minimized by maintaining the patient in a neutral thermal environment. Since renal function may be impaired, careful fluid and electrolyte management is critical.

D. AIRWAY MANAGEMENT

1. Position the infant to allow slight hyperextension of the head. Periodic rotation from supine to lateral position promotes tracheobronchial drainage.

2. Tracheal suctioning is usually necessary to remove thick secretions during the exudative phase, which begins at about 48 hours of age.

E. OXYGEN ADMINISTRATION

Warmed, humidified, oxygen-enriched gas mixtures are delivered into small lucite hoods placed over the infant's head or via endotracheal tubes to maintain the Pa_{O_2} between 50 and 80 torr.

F. VASCULAR CATHETERS

1. Place umbilical arterial catheter in infants requiring an $F_{I_{O_2}}$ of 0.4 or greater for arterial blood gas (ABG) and BP monitoring.

2. An umbilical venous catheter may be placed into the central circulation for central venous pressure (CVP) monitoring.

G. HYPOVOLEMIA AND ANEMIA

1. Measure central hematocrit and BP serially beginning as soon after birth as practical.

2. During the acute phase of the illness maintain the hematocrit reading at 40% to 50% by transfusion.

3. During resolution, hematocrit readings greater than 30% should suffice.

H. ACIDOSIS

1. Metabolic acidosis (a base deficit of 6 mEq/L or greater) requires evaluation for the possible causes, which include hypovolemia, hypoxia, sequelae of asphyxia, or hypothermia, infection, CNS hemorrhage, renal tubular defects, and metabolic disease.

2. Empirical attempts to correct base deficits of 6 to 9 mEq/L with blood transfusion, albumin infusion, or diluted sodium bicarbonate ($NaHCO_3$) are recommended if the pH is less than 7.25. Sodium bicarbonate treatment requires adequate ventilation to be effective.

3. Base deficits of 10 to 12 mEq/L or greater are usually treated even if the pH is above 7.25.

4. Dose of sodium bicarbonate (mEq) = base deficit × body weight in kg × 0.3. Assess effect with ABG.

5. Administer bicarbonate slowly as a 0.5 mEq/L solution.

6. A *pure* respiratory acidosis level in the range of 7.20 to 7.30 may be tolerable. When the pH falls below 7.20 on a respiratory basis, assisted ventilation is recommended.

I. FEEDING

1. Attempt to start gastric feeding via orogastric tube between 48 and 72 hours of age, if the cardiovascular system is stable and pulmonary disease is under appropriate management.

2. Avoid nipple feeding in infants with respiratory rates above 70 per minute to minimize the risk of aspiration.

3. Begin parenteral nutrition if enteral feeding will be delayed.

J. ROENTGENOGRAPHIC STUDIES

Roentgenographic studies are used for the following:

1. To diagnose and assess the course of the disease.

2. To document the position of endotracheal tubes, chest tubes, and umbilical catheters.

3. To detect complications such as pneumothorax, pneumopericardium, and necrotizing enterocolitis.

K. COAGULATION

1. Give vitamin K oxide immediately after birth, and weekly in infants receiving antibiotics and while receiving no enteral feeding.

2. Monitor prothrombin time (PT), partial thromboplastin time (PTT), and platelet counts.

L. IRRITABILITY

1. The Pa_{O_2} and Pa_{CO_2} of sick newborns may be adversely affected by struggling and agitation. Handle these infants gently and only as frequently as necessary.

2. Occasionally, morphine sulfate or pancuronium bromide may be indicated in infants on ventilators who cannot be soothed.

M. INFECTION

1. Most infants with respiratory distress deserve evaluation for sepsis and pneumonia and initial coverage with antibiotics until culture results are known.

2. Group B β-hemolytic *Streptococcus* infection may mimic RDS clinically and roentgenographically.

N. SUDDEN DETERIORATION IN CLINICAL CONDITION MAY BE DUE TO THE FOLLOWING:

1. Alveolar rupture and the development of pulmonary interstitial emphysema (PIE) and/or pneumothorax or pneumopericardium. Recognition and treatment of tension pneumothorax are outlined in section V.

2. Loss of continuity of the oxygen delivery or ventilatory system.

a. Make sure that connections in the oxygen and pressure delivery systems are secure.

b. Obstruction of the endotracheal tube, accidental extubation, or advancement of the endotracheal tube into the right main-stem bronchus can often be detected by assessment of the tube position and function.

c. When in doubt about obstruction of endotracheal tubes or accidental extubation, remove the tube, and ventilate the infant with a bag and mask. The endotracheal tube can be replaced when the infant's condition is stabilized.

3. These less common conditions may cause sudden deterioration: intracranial hemorrhage, septic shock, hypoglycemia, kernicterus, transient hyperammonemia, or inherited metabolic disorders.

O. PATENT DUCTUS ARTERIOSUS

1. When RDS is very severe, a *right-to-left* shunt may occur through the ductus (see section IV. **Pulmonary Hypertension**).

2. With improvement in respiratory function, pulmonary vascular resistance may fall dramatically, allowing a *left-to-right* ductal shunt. Clinical features may include the following:

a. A systolic heart murmur.

b. Widening of the pulse pressure.

c. Carbon dioxide retention.

d. Apnea and abdominal distention.

e. Failure to progress in withdrawing ventilatory support.

P. MANAGEMENT OF RESPIRATORY FAILURE IN RDS

1. The decision to *intervene* in RDS with pulmonary support techniques other than supplemental oxygen should be documented in the chart according to the criteria in Table 13–1.

2. For infants weighing less than 1,500 gm, trials of CPAP may cause unwarranted expenditures of energy (by infant, nurse, and physician).

3. Initially, we manipulate the ventilator in such fashion that inspired oxygen can be reduced to an FI_{O_2} of 0.6 to 0.8. This usually happens promptly once a mean airway pressure of 12 to 14 mm Hg has been achieved.

TABLE 13–1.—CRITERIA FOR INTERVENTION WITH PULMONARY SUPPORT TECHNIQUES

INDICATIONS FOR INTERVENTION			THERAPY
AGE (HR)	Pao_2 (TORR)	FI_{O_2}	
<24	<50	.65	Noninvasive*
	<50	.80	CPAP via ET
	<50	.80	Mechanical ventilation
>24	<50	.80	Noninvasive*
	<50	1.00	CPAP via ET
	<50	1.00	Mechanical ventilation (may follow trial of CPAP)

*Noninvasive techniques include nasal CPAP, head box CPAP, or CNP. These techniques are usually not successful for infants weighing less than 1,500 gm, and usually we do not recommend them for such infants.

OTHER INDICATIONS FOR MECHANICAL VENTILATION include a $Paco_2$ level greater than 60 torr, apnea, and resuscitation.

CPAP indicates continuous positive airway pressure; CNP indicates continuous negative pressure.

a. Unless the Pa_{O_2} is greater than 100 torr, oxygen concentrations are lowered by small increments, or about 5% (e.g., from 65% to 60%).

b. The effect of change in settings is assessed by blood gas analysis ten to 15 minutes following the change.

c. At low concentrations, inspired oxygen (e.g., less than 40% oxygen) decrements of 2% to 3% may be appropriate.

4. The second objective is to reduce inspiratory pressures to prevent pulmonary barotrauma.

a. In general, if the Fl_{O_2} is above 0.6, reduce inspired oxygen.

b. If Fl_{O_2} is between 0.4 and 0.6, reduce the parameter that is considered most hazardous to the patient.

c. When the Fl_{O_2} reaches 0.4, the major emphasis should be to reduce inspiratory and end-expiratory pressures.

d. Extubation is usually accomplished when the Fl_{O_2} is between 0.3 and 0.4.

5. Carbon dioxide retention may occur during the acute phase of RDS. When therapeutic attempts to correct this abnormality adversely affect oxygenation, consult the neonatal fellow or attending physician.

Q. SURVIVAL

Consult Table 13–2.

II. RDS TYPE II, TRANSIENT TACHYPNEA, AND RETAINED LUNG FLUID SYNDROMES

A. EARLY CLINICAL COURSE

The early clinical course resembles RDS, but the chest x-ray film shows hilar streaking, fluid in the minor fissure, and increased vascular and interstitial markings.

B. ETIOLOGY

1. Failure to clear the pulmonary fluid present at birth or, equally likely, a failure of the lung to stop producing lung fluid at the intrauterine rate.

TABLE 13–2.—UCDMC
RDS SURVIVAL, 1977–1981*

BIRTH WEIGHT (GM)	SURVIVAL, NO. (%)	
<750	35	(29)
751–1,000	81	(53)
1,001–1,250	85	(68)
1,251–1,500	77	(88)
1,501–1,750	58	(91)
1,751–2,000	61	(93)
>2,001	123	(97)

*Includes 371 infants treated with mechanical ventilations, 29 CPAP and O_2, and 120 with supplemental O_2 only. University of California, Davis Medical Center indicates.

2. Frequently observed in the following:

a. Intrapartum asphyxia.

b. Excessive maternal medication.

c. Cesarean section.

d. Infants of diabetic mothers.

C. TRANSIENT TACHYPNEA

Transient tachypnea of the newborn is associated with an essentially normal chest x-ray film and may be the mildest form of the above disorder.

1. In transient tachypnea, there is little, if any, requirement for supplemental oxygen.

2. Hypocarbia is often present.

D. COURSE AND THERAPY

1. Rarely, clinical course is severe and similar to RDS.

2. Most infants improve dramatically by 24 to 48 hours.

3. Therapy is aimed at correcting pulmonary insufficiency by the least invasive techniques possible and avoiding iatrogenic problems.

III. MECONIUM ASPIRATION

Ten percent to 15% of newborn infants have passed meconium before birth. Three percent to 5% of these aspirate meconium. While potentially fatal pulmonary failure may accompany meconium aspiration, controversy exists about the etiology of the pulmonary insufficiency since long-standing hypertrophy of pulmonary vascular smooth muscle has been observed in fatal cases. However, if airway obstruction plays a role, this aspect may be preventable and treatment for this condition should begin in the delivery room. Fetal asphyxia is common in either case.

A. RECOGNITION Communication between obstetrics and neonatology after recognition of meconium-stained amniotic fluid is essential.

B. PHARYNGEAL SUCTIONING As soon as the head is delivered, meconium is cleared from the nose and pharynx by the obstetrician.

C. TRACHEAL SUCTION Visualize and suction the trachea under direct vision immediately after birth.

1. A No. 10 French Argyle suction catheter is suitable for the infant with spontaneous respirations.

2. When resuscitation is anticipated, intubate immediately and suction the trachea before ventilating. Use oxygen-enriched gas for ventilating.

3. Mouth-to-tube suction during withdrawal of the endotracheal tube may be necessary, in some instances, to remove thick meconium.

4. When in doubt, intubate and suction.

D. TRACHEAL LAVAGE

1. If NO meconium is suctioned from the trachea, stabilize patient and transport to intensive care nursery for observation and chest x-ray.

2. If meconium is suctioned from the trachea, ventilate for one to 3 minutes and then instill 1 to 2 ml of sterile saline into the endotracheal tube. After a spontaneous breath or a brief puff on the ventilating bag, suction the tube and again ventilate for one to three minutes. Repeat saline lavages several times or until clear. Extubate if spontaneous respirations are adequate.

   a. Transport to intensive care nursery for immediate chest x-ray (look for infiltrate, pneumothorax, or both) and intensive care observation.

   b. If infiltrate is present on x-ray film or signs of respiratory distress develop, begin percussion, vibration, and suction every three to four hours. Ultrasonic mist may be beneficial during the first 12 to 24 hours after birth.

   c. Have a 20 to 30-ml syringe with a three-way stopcock and needle present at the bedside for emergency treatment of pneumothorax.

   d. Oxygen therapy should be guided by blood gases.

E. FEEDING   Delay oral feeding as long as the respiratory rate is above 70 per minute.

F. CORTICOSTEROIDS AND ANTIBIOTICS   The values of corticosteroids and antibiotics are controversial. Consult the attending neonatologist.

IV. PULMONARY HYPERTENSION IN THE NEWBORN

This entity is also referred to as persistent fetal circulation (PFC). Pulmonary hypertension in the newborn may lead to RIGHT-to-LEFT shunting through the foramen ovale, ductus arteriosus, or both. Severe hypoxemia may occur. When it is due to intense pulmonary vasospasm of normal, or thickened, arteriolar smooth muscle, therapy with hyperventilation, vasodilator drugs, or both may be lifesaving. Fatal cases seem to have a marked increase in pulmonary vascular smooth muscle or marked decrease in the number of small pulmonary arteries, i.e., pulmonary hypoplasia.

A. CLINICAL FEATURES

1. Pulmonary hypertension occurs in term or post-term infants without lung disease and at any gestational age as a complication of pulmonary disease. It occurs frequently in the following instances:

   a. Meconium aspiration

   b. Congenital pneumonia

   c. Severe RDS

   d. Diaphragmatic hernia

   e. Chromosomal disorders

2. Pulmonary vasospasm may be responsible for the "flip-flop" phenomenon sometimes seen during the acute phase of RDS (e.g., a marked decrease in Pao_2 following a small decrement in oxygen concentration or ventilator pressure).

3. The course varies from mild (with spontaneous resolution) to death from intractable hypoxia.

4. Duration of illness rarely exceeds one week.

B. DIAGNOSIS

1. Suspect when the clinical severity of pulmonary insufficiency is greater than the roentgenographic findings suggest.

2. Suspect when pulmonary insufficiency is refractory to ventilatory therapy, e.g., increased inspiratory pressures and positive end-expiratory pressure.

3. Electrocardiograph is usually normal.

4. Echocardiographic evidence of pulmonary hypertension, right-to-left atrial shunt, and absence of structural heart disease (essential for diagnosis) is usually present. Left ventricular dysfunction is also noted in some cases.

5. Simultaneous right radial or temporal artery and aortic Pa_{O_2} with difference of 10 torr or greater (ductal shunt). This is not present when the shunt is primarily at the atrial level or when the ductus is closed.

6. Positive response to therapy with hyperventilation or tolazoline.

C. MANAGEMENT   Therapy is aimed at promoting pulmonary vasodilation.

1. Hypoxemia, acidosis, hypercapnia, hypoglycemia, hypocalcemia, hyperviscosity, and systemic hypotension should all be corrected.

2. Hyperventilation producing a Pa_{CO_2} less than 30 and a pH greater than 7.50 is often associated with dramatic increases in the Pa_{O_2}.

a. The mechanism of action of hyperventilation as a pulmonary vasodilator is currently unknown.

b. Not all infants with severe lung disease can be hyperventilated.

c. Complications of hyperventilation have primarily been pulmonary air leaks.

d. Decreased coronary and cerebral blood flow and hypocalcemic tetany have not been reported secondary to hyperventilation alkalosis in infants.

3. Pharmacologic pulmonary vasodilator therapy should only be given after consultation with a neonatal fellow or attending. We usually use tolazoline, but other vasodilators may be used in some centers.

a. Infuse bolus of tolazoline, 1 to 2 mg/kg, over ten minutes via scalp vein or arm vein.

b. Monitor BP continuously and be prepared to treat systemic hypotension with volume or dopamine.

c. Monitor arterial blood gases at 0, 30, and 60 minutes in relation to time of administration of tolazoline.

d. If patient does not exhibit cutaneous flushing, repeat bolus dose.

e. Begin tolazoline infusion in scalp vein at rate of 2 mg/kg/hr.

f. A positive response is an abrupt rise in Pa_{O_2} of 15 torr or greater (usually 50 to 100 torr).

g. Increase tolazoline infusion rate (up to 4 to 6 mg/kg/hr) as indicated by blood gas analysis.

h. When $F_{I_{O_2}}$ can be reduced to 0.6, begin to decrease tolazoline infusion rate.

i. Complications
    i. Systemic hypotension
    ii. Hypertension
    iii. Gastric distention
    iv. GI tract bleeding
    v. Transient renal failure

4. Adjunctive Therapy

a. Sedation or paralysis may facilitate hyperventilation.

b. Dopamine, 2.5 to 10.0 μg/kg/min, may support cardiac output when left ventricular dysfunction is present.

c. Extracorporeal membrane oxygenators (ECMO) may prove to be useful in severe and refractory cases.

5. Outcome

a. About 75% of affected term infants survive.

b. About 75% of the survivors are developmentally and neurologically normal.

V. EXTRAPULMONARY AIR

Alveolar rupture, with extrapulmonary collection of air, may occur spontaneously or as a complication of ventilatory therapy in newborns. After alveolar rupture, air may accumulate in the interstitial spaces (pulmonary interstitial emphysema [PIE]) or it may dissect along bronchovascular channels to the hilum. Rupture of mediastinal walls leads to a pneumomediastinum, pneumothorax, or both. Accumulation of air in the intrapleural space may cause minimal to severe embarrassment of pulmonary function. While spontaneous pneumothorax occurs in 1% to 2% of "normal" newborns, the incidence is higher in the presence of pulmonary disease and considerably higher when ventilatory assistance is required (15% to 25%). Air may also dissect into the pericardium (pneumopericardium) and lead to cardiac tamponade. Dissection of gas into the peritoneum, while uncommon, is usually benign but may lead to a mistaken diagnosis of intestinal perforation.

A. SIGNS OF TENSION PNEUMOTHORAX

1. Sudden clinical or blood gas deterioration with signs of respiratory distress (cyanosis, tachypnea, retractions).

2. Shift of the apical cardiac impulse *(most consistent finding)*.

3. Decreased breath sounds unilaterally, or bilaterally, possibly accompanied by a bulging or prominence of the chest on that side. **NOTE:** Absent breath sounds on right side or both sides could be due to an endotracheal tube in right mainstem bronchus or a plugged endotracheal tube.

4. Abdominal distention with sudden descent of liver or spleen.

5. Differential resonance to percussion on right vs. left.

6. Acute increase in systolic BP followed by narrowing of pulse pressure.

B. DIAGNOSIS

1. Physical findings as above.

2. Chest x-ray film.

3. Transillumination of the chest.

4. Diagnostic and therapeutic thoracentesis.

C. MANAGEMENT

1. **Asymptomatic or Mildly Symptomatic Pneumothorax**
   a. Close observation.
   b. Supplemental oxygen to maintain Pa_{O_2} at 80 to 100 torr.

2. **Symptomatic Pneumothorax**   chest tube to water seal suction (– 10 cm water) or Heimlich valve.

3. **Imminent Demise**   Emergency thoracentesis.

D. PNEUMOMEDIASTINUM RARELY REQUIRES TREATMENT

E. PNEUMOPERICARDIUM IS OFTEN LIFE-THREATENING

1. Shock secondary to tamponade usually has a sudden onset.

2. Pericardial drainage via needle aspiration, placement of a pericardial drainage tube, or both is usually necessary.

3. On occasion, a pneumopericardium causes relatively few symptoms and disappears spontaneously.

VI. CHRONIC LUNG DISEASE OF PREMATURITY

Chronic lung disease is a disturbing and confusing sequela of extreme prematurity, oxygen and ventilatory therapy, and possibly patent ductus arteriosus. Some form of chronic lung disease occurs in approximately 15% of premature infants requiring mechanical ventilation for pulmonary insufficiency. There is significant mortality and considerable morbidity (long-term dependence on oxygen and prolonged hospitalization) from these conditions. However, full recovery of lung function usually occurs in the survivors anywhere from a few months to 3 years of age. There is confusion because of the variety of names applied to these syndromes and whether or not they are distinct entities or continuum of a single disorder.

A. CHRONIC LUNG DISEASE FOLLOWING VENTILATORY THERAPY FOR RDS: BRONCHOPULMONARY DYSPLASIA (BPD)

1. Following the acute phase of RDS, failure to improve is noted. At 10 to 14 days of age these infants may begin to increase their oxygen requirements.

2. Carbon dioxide retention is routinely observed.

3. A stable oxygen requirement supervenes at 3 to 4 weeks of age.

4. Resolution is slow, requiring one to six months or longer for the infant to tolerate breathing room air.

5. Chest x-ray varies from a cystic, bubbly appearance in the severe forms to a streaky, fibrotic appearance in the less involved. Hyperinflation is routinely present.

6. These infants are predisposed to pneumonia for at least the first year of life.

7. Mortality may approach 30%. Death often occurs beyond the neonatal period, between 1 and 12 months of age.

B. DIURETIC-RESPONSIVE INTERSTITIAL PNEUMONOPATHY (DRIP)

1. Low fluctuating oxygen requirement follows resolution of RDS.

2. Chest x-ray fails to clear completely and there is a haze or "veil" possibly due to mild diffuse atelectasis, interstitial edema, or both.

3. Pulmonary function improves with vigorous diuretic therapy (furosemide in doses of 1 to 4 mg/kg and one to three times per day).

4. Usually resolves by 4 to 6 weeks of age.

C. WILSON-MIKITY SYNDROME

1. This uncommon syndrome is seen in small premature infants who initially have nearly normal chest x-ray and minimal respiratory difficulty.

2. Pulmonary insufficiency develops between 4 and 35 days of age.

3. Chest x-ray film shows multiple cystic lesions; hyperaeration alternating with a coarse thickening of interstitial structure (honey-comb lung).

4. Nearly half of these infants die. The survivors have normal chest x-ray films and lung function by 1 to 2 years of age.

D. CHRONIC PULMONARY INSUFFICIENCY OF PREMATURITY (CPIP)

1. Delayed form, with onset at 4 to 7 days.

2. Infants weigh less than 1,250 gm, with no early lung pathological signs.

3. Chest x-ray seldom shows more than a diffuse haze.

4. Oxygen requirements persist for two to four weeks. Recovery is usually complete by 60 days of age.

5. Apneic spells and need for supplemental oxygen are early signs.

6. Mortality is said to be 10% to 20% as a result of this condition.

E. MANAGEMENT

1. No specific therapy exists for any of these conditions.

2. Supportive therapy often includes oxygen and ventilatory assistance.

3. Hematocrit reading should be maintained above 35%.

4. Nutritional goal is to provide maximum calories with minimal sodium and free water required for normal renal function.

5. Few of these infants tolerate normal fluid intake; fluid overload and pulmonary edema are frequently observed. Diuretics are frequently helpful.

6. Weight changes and serum electrolyte levels must be carefully monitored.

7. Chronic cor pulmonale may lead to trial of digitalis therapy.

8. Corticosteroids, usually prednisone (2.5 mg/kg twice a day), may improve lung function in some infants. Dramatic improvement should occur in two to four days. If this is not observed, stop prednisone administration. If improvement does occur, a ten-day course is given.

9. Theophylline has been helpful in some infants beyond 6 weeks of age with carbon dioxide retention, especially when wheezing has been noted. Be sure to monitor blood levels when this drug is used.

10. N-acetyl-L-cysteine nebulization may be helpful in some infants with recurrent atelectasis due to increased pulmonary secretions.

11. Prophylactic chest physiotherapy is usually prescribed once or twice a day.

14

Neonatal Apnea

Approximately 25% of infants weighing less than 1,800 gm at birth will have at least one apneic episode during their nursery course. The associated bradycardia and hypoxemia may be life threatening. Intermittent periodic breathing is common and must be differentiated from apnea.

A. DEFINITION

1. **Apnea** "Cessation of breathing for 20 seconds or longer, or a briefer episode associated with bradycardia, cyanosis, or pallor" (AAP Task Force).

2. **Periodic Breathing** Respiratory pauses of five to ten seconds with normal respirations between episodes not associated with bradycardia, but may coincide with hypoxemia.

B. CAUSES Apnea is not a disease, but a symptom.

1. Decreased Tissue Oxygen Delivery

a. Hypoxemia

b. Anemia

c. Heart failure

2. Pulmonary Disease With Decreased Lung Compliance

a. RDS, pneumonia, etc.

b. PDA with increased pulmonary blood flow

c. Hypoinflation or hyperinflation during or after ventilation therapy

3. Feeding Related (Vagal Mediated)

a. Nasogastric tube passage; gastric distention

b. Gastroesophageal reflux

4. Airway Obstruction

a. Excessive oral secretions

b. Anatomic obstruction

5. Sepsis—Bacterial or Viral

6. Convulsive   Cardiac rate is usually maintained during the seizure

7. Metabolic Imbalance

a. Hypoglycemia

b. Electrolyte imbalance

c. Lactic acidosis

8. Environmental Temperature Fluctuations   This is more common with rising environmental temperatures.

9. CNS Hemorrhage or Abnormalities

10. Drug Induced   (Usually maternally administered)

11. Prematurity   All other causes should be excluded before making this diagnosis.

a. Respiratory drive immaturity
  i. Symptoms mostly begin in first two weeks of life.

b. Prolonged sleep—more common during REM sleep
  i. REM sleep is more frequent in premature infants.
  ii. Premature infants sleep 80% to 90% of the time.
  iii. Ventilatory response to hypoxia is more sustained in non–REM sleep.

C. EVALUATION

All infants who weigh less than 1,500 gm at birth and larger infants at risk should have cardiorespiratory monitoring for at least ten days or until mature respiratory control is documented.

1. History and Physical Examination

a. Attempt to characterize frequency, duration, and temporal associations of events.

b. Notation of association with bradycardia.

2. First Event or Acute Onset

a. Oxygenation and ventilation
  i. Arterial blood gas measurements.
  ii. Transcutaneous pO_2 and pCO_2 monitoring.

b. Sepsis work-up, including CBC count, chest x-ray film, electrolyte measurement, and metabolic screen.

3. CNS Evaluation

a. EEG, asleep and awake

b. Cranial ultrasound or CT scan

c. Brain-stem auditory evoked potentials

4. Cardiac Evaluation

a. ECG

b. Echocardiography

5. Gastrointestinal Tract

a. Cardiorespiratory activity with feeding

b. Fluoroscopy or bronchoscopy as indicated.

c. Esophageal pH with history of esophageal reflux

d. Radionuclide scan after feeding marker

6. Pneumogram, Somnogram, or Polygraphic Sleep Study

a. Depending on ability of laboratory, many of the above studies can be incorporated into the polygraphic study.

D. THERAPY   should be aimed at eliminating the primary cause.

1. Specific Therapy to Treat

Hypoxemia, PDA, anemia, metabolic aberrations, sepsis, gastroesophageal reflux, seizure activity.

2. Symptomatic Treatment

a. Tactile stimulation—cutaneous

b. Vestibular stimulation—"bump beds"

c. Decrease environmental temperature to low neutral thermal environment

d. Mechanical ventilation for severe cases

3. Pharmacologic Agents for Apnea of Prematurity

a. Theophylline, loading dose of 5 to 6 mg/kg IV or orally, then 2 to 3 mg/kg every 8 hours. Follow levels after the third to fourth dose and observe the infant for tachycardia and emesis.

b. Caffeine citrate, loading dose of 20 mg/kg orally, then 5 to 10 mg/kg/day in one or two daily doses.

c. A lower incidence of side effects seems to be associated with caffeine. However, blood levels are not routinely available.

E. CRITERIA FOR HOME MONITORING

1. The patient is ready to be discharged except for the following:

a. Documented apnea without treatable cause or with inadequate response to therapy.

b. Abnormal pneumogram or polygraphic sleep study.

c. Family history of two or more siblings with sudden infant death syndrome.

d. Potential airway obstruction or chronic hypoxemia.

2. Consider family psychological stress, medical/legal aspects, and use of correct monitor type.

a. All care providers should have CPR training.

b. Monitor type should be cardiorespiratory, not apnea pad.

F. INDICATIONS FOR DISCONTINUANCE OF HOME MONITOR

1. No clinical apnea for two months.

2. No apnea requiring stimulation for three months.

3. Normal pneumogram or polygraphic sleep study.

4. Infant must have experienced stress of nasopharyngitis or immunizations without recurrence of symptoms.

REFERENCES

1. Rigatto H. Apnea. *Pediatr. Clin North Am.* 29:1105, 1983.
2. Aranda J.V., Grondin D., Sasyniuk B.I.: Pharmacologic considerations in the therapy of neonatal apnea. *Pediatr. Clin North Am.* 28:113–133, 1981.
3. Relationship between apnea and bradycardia in preterm infant. *Acta Paed. Scand.* 70:785, 1981.
4. Kattwinkel J.: Neonatal apnea: Pathogenesis and therapy. *J. Pediatr.* 90:342–347, 1977.

15

Shock and Hypoperfusion

"Shock" in the newborn may present as hypotension or hypoperfusion with normal BP. Etiologic considerations as well as the therapeutic approach vary with the postnatal age of the infant and with the clinical setting.

A. CLASSIFICATION

1. Hypovolemic

   a. Blood loss may be external (including fetal-maternal, placental transfusions) or internal.

   b. Plasma loss may accompany major abdominal surgery.

   c. Extracellular fluid loss due to vomiting, diarrhea, or high insensible water loss.

2. Cardiogenic

   a. Sequelae of severe asphyxia, hypoglycemia, acidemia, congenital heart disease, or myocardial dysfunction (IDMs, myocarditis).

   b. End stage of other forms of shock.

3. Distributive   (Usually septic shock).

B. ASSESSMENT

1. Physical Examination   emphasizing cardiopulmonary status, edema, peripheral circulation, BP, and site of infection.

2. Basic monitoring

   a. Blood pressure using Doppler or preferably arterial line.

   b. Monitor urine output, input/output carefully (bladder catheterization is desirable in severe cases), and weights.

c. Arterial blood gases to assess for acidosis or hypoxemia.

d. Central venous pressure is often useful and occasionally critical for management. This may be measured by an umbilical venous catheter above the diagram or by a catheter placed via the external jugular or peripheral vein.

e. Aortic diastolic time constant (τ) may be useful in assessing systemic vascular resistance.

f. Serially monitor neutrophil count, platelet count, and clotting factors.

3. Indicators of Blood Volume (or Effective Blood Volume)

a. Change in hematocrit readings.

b. Response to a fluid challenge of 10 ml/kg of saline (monitor BP, CVP, and urine output).

c. Betke-Kleihauer acid elution test on mother if fetal-maternal transfusion is suspected.

4. Indicators of Cardiac Function

a. Assessment of cardiopulmonary patterns and other vital organ functions, BP, and perfusion.

b. Echocardiogram: anatomical defects, myocardial function (systolic time intervals, left ventricle (LV) ejection fraction, left ventricular end diastolic (LVED) and systolic (LVES) pressures, and atrial bubble study).

c. ECG, CVP, and diastolic pressure analysis.

5. Indicators of Septic Shock

a. Evidence or proof of sepsis.

b. Hypoperfusion usually prominent, often with normal central BP.

c. Capillary leak of protein and fluid with edema or sclerema.

d. Oliguria, proteinuria, with or without hypotension.

e. Pulmonary hypertension with persistence of fetal circulation is common.

C. TREATMENT

1. Increase the Blood Volume and Red Cell Mass to maintain BP and to maximize oxygen content. Use BP, CVP,

peripheral infusion, and metabolic acidosis as guides to volume to be transfused.

2. **Maximize Cardiac Output** Inotropes should be introduced early in septic shock, where there is evidence of oliguria, hypotension, or acidosis.

   a. Dopamine, 5 to 10 μg/kg/min IV.

   b. Dobutamine, 5 to 10 μg/kg/min may be added concurrently. Experience in newborns is limited.

   c. Digitalis should be used selectively, and may be hazardous in face of hypoxia or toxic myocardiopathy.

3. **Maximize Oxygenation** Tolazoline may be useful when pulmonary hypertension produces hypoxemia. In septic shock, tolazoline should be used cautiously and in conjunction with inotropic agents and volume expansion, since systemic hypotension is likely.

D. CONTROVERSIAL THERAPIES

1. **Corticosteroids** may prevent adrenal insufficiency, stabilize lysosomal membranes, and inhibit complement-induced granulocyte aggregation. Massive doses with 2 to 6 mg/kg of dexamethasone every four to six hours have been advocated in the early stage of disease.

2. **Indomethacin** which inhibits cyclooxygenase activity and potentiates lipoxygenase activity, may block pulmonary artery pressure changes in experimental septic shock.

3. **Naloxone** which competitively inhibits effects of endorphins, may be effective in experimental hemorrhagic and endotoxic shock.

4. **Exchange Transfusion** may be effective in scleremic septic newborns and probably effective in group B β-hemolytic streptococcal sepsis when a donor with type-specific antibody is identified.

5. **Leukocyte Transfusion** may be effective in patients with severe neutropenia and bone marrow depression. Use of irradiated buffy coat concentrates is preferable.

16

Evaluation of Cyanosis in the Newborn

Cyanosis in the newborn should be considered a medical emergency and should be approached in a fast and efficient way. Once cyanosis is confirmed by an arterial blood gas measurement demonstrating a low Pao_2, the basic question is whether it is cardiac or pulmonary in origin.

A. DIAGNOSIS

1. The mechanism of pulmonary cyanosis can be alveolar hypoventilation (e.g., CNS), impaired diffusion (i.e., pneumonia), right-to-left intrapulmonary shunt, ventilation perfusion inequality (e.g., atelectasis), or red cell impairment (e.g., methemoglobinemia).

2. Table 16–1 presents a diagnostic approach to the cyanotic newborn. Physical examination, chest x-ray film, and simple laboratory tests should differentiate major causes of cyanosis.

3. A differential diagnosis of the most common cyanotic cardiac lesions of the newborn can be seen in Table 16–2.

4. If congenital heart disease or persistence of fetal circulation (PFC) is suspected, immediate consultation with a pediatric cardiologist is indicated.

B. MANAGEMENT

Most babies with cyanotic heart disease are candidates for surgical correction. Appropriate supportive measures improve the ultimate outcome.

TABLE 16-1.—SCREENING OF THE CYANOTIC NEWBORN

QUESTION	CLINICAL OBSERVATIONS	LABORATORY TESTS	ANSWER
Is cyanosis central?	Blue tongue and mucosa		Yes
Is cyanosis due to noncardiac or pulmonary reasons?		Normal P_{O_2}, increased hematocrit and hemoglobin values	Polycythemia
		Normal P_{O_2}, decreased blood glucose level	Hypoglycemia
Is cyanosis cardiac or pulmonary?	Respiratory distress (retractions)	Decreased P_{O_2}, increased P_{CO_2}, 10 min 100% F_{IO_2}, P_{O_2} >100 mm Hg	Pulmonary
	Tachypnea	Decreased P_{O_2}, normal P_{CO_2}, 10 min 100% F_{IO_2}, P_{O_2} unchanged	Cardiac
Is cyanosis due to congenital heart disease or persistent fetal circulation?	Tachypnea	10 min 100% F_{IO_2}, P_{O_2} 50–100 mm Hg, Umbilical artery P_{O_2} at least 10 mm Hg less than right radial P_{O_2}	Persistent fetal circulation

TABLE 16–2.—DIFFERENTIAL DIAGNOSIS OF MORE COMMON CYANOTIC HEART LESIONS*

LESION	PHYSICAL SIGNS	CHEST X-RAY	ECG	ECHOCARDIOGRAM
Transposition of great vessels	Single S-2, occasionally systolic murmurs	Egg-shaped heart, increased vasculature	RVH	Aorta coming off RV, MPA coming off LV
Truncus arteriosus	Often systolic ejection click; usually single S-2, systolic murmur; Rarely early diastolic	Increased vascularity, occasionally egg-shaped heart	CVH	Truncus overriding septum, pulmonary artery coming off main truncus
Total anomalous venous return	Occasionally widely split S-2	Pulmonary venous congestion, occasionally "snowman" appearance	RVH	Double echo behind LA

Hypoplastic right heart (tricuspid atresia, pulmonary atresia)	Single S-2, occasionally systolic murmurs	Decreased pulmonary vascularity, cardiomegaly in cases of severe TI	LAD, LVH or LV predominance	Evidence of atretic tricuspid or pulmonary valves, small RV
Fallot's tetralogy variants (severe outflow stenosis obstruction)	Single S-2, occasionally murmurs	Boot-shaped heart, decreased vascularity	RVH	Overriding aorta, stenotic RV outflow
Ebstein's anomaly	Occasionally split S-1, systolic murmurs of TI	Severe cardiomegaly, decreased vascularity	RAH RVH Conduction defect	Large RA Small RV

*TI indicates tricuspid insufficiency; RVH, right ventricular hypertrophy; CVH, combined ventricular hypertrophy; LAD, left atrial diameter; LVH, left ventricular hypertrophy; RAH, right atrial hypertrophy; RV, right ventricle; MPA, main pulmonary artery; LV, left ventricle; LA, left atrium.

1. Correct metabolic acidosis, hypoglycemia, and hypocalcemia.

2. Oxygen.

3. Transfusion: Aim to raise the hematocrit reading above 45%.

4. Prostaglandin E_1 (0.1 μ/kg/min IV) is indicated for all ductal dependent obstructive lesions and, according to some investigators, for all cyanotic lesions short term.

5. Palliative invasive procedures, i.e., balloon atrial septostomy.

6. Palliative surgery, i.e., aortopulmonary shunts.

17

Congestive Heart Failure in the Newborn

Heart failure is defined as inadequate cardiac output for the needs of the body (Table 17–1). The general pathogenic mechanisms involve increased preload, increased afterload, impaired contractility, and chronotropic abnormalities.

The newborn myocardium has a poor response to pressure and volume loads because of immaturity of contractile elements and sympathetic innervation. Congestive heart failure in the newborn is not expressed as pure right or left failure as in the adult, but with mixed symptoms from both sides.

A. PHYSICAL FINDINGS

1. Increased rate and depth of respirations, coughing, wheezes, and rales.

2. Tachycardia, active precordium, muffled heart sounds, murmurs, and gallop rhythm.

3. Abnormal pulses

   a. Bounding (PDA or AV malformation).

   b. Weak peripheral pulses in general (hypoplastic left heart).

   c. Normal pulses in upper extremities, absent pulses in lower extremities (coarctation).

4. Hepatosplenomegaly, rarely edema, mottling, pallor, sweating.

5. Difficult feeding and failure to thrive.

B. DIAGNOSTIC STUDIES

1. Chest x-ray film

a. Heart size—look for cardiomegaly and specific chamber enlargement.

b. Vascularity—increased vascularity is evidence of pulmonary venous congestion or increased pulmonary blood flow.

c. Aortic arch, position.

2. ECG (See ECG section)

a. Rhythm, rate (sinus tachycardia, paroxysmal atrial tachycardia [PAT] heart block).

b. Mean frontal (QRS) axis.

c. P waves for right atrial hypertrophy (Ebstein's anomaly, transient tricuspid insufficiency) and left atrial hypertrophy (left-to-right shunt).

d. RV hypertrophy most common or combined ventricular hypertrophy or LV predominance (rarely).

e. ST-T wave changes—in transient myocardial ischemia, severe aortic stenosis, or LV strain.

3. Echocardiogram (See Echocardiogram section)

a. Morphologic information—diagnosis of hypoplastic left heart syndrome, coarctation, ventricular septal defect (VSD), transposition, truncus, etc.

b. Physiologic information—shortening fraction or ejection fraction of the LV and RV.

c. Systolic time intervals for both main pulmonary artery and aorta.

TABLE 17–1.—COMMON CAUSES OF HEART FAILURE IN INFANCY

1st day of life	Transient myocardial ischemia
	Cardiomyopathy (infants of diabetic mothers)
	Massive tricuspid insufficiency
	Massive pulmonary insufficiency
2nd day to 1st week	Hypoplastic left heart syndrome
	Coarctation of the aorta
1st to 4th week	Ventricular septal defect
	Patent ductus arteriosus

    d. Quantitation of shunts, cardiac output, and valvular insufficiency by Doppler echocardiography.

4. Laboratory Chemistry Studies

    a. Hemoglobin, hematocrit, blood glucose, electrolytes, calcium, and urine analysis.

    b. Blood gases.

C. MANAGEMENT

1. Maintenance of Neutral Thermal Environment and Metabolic Homeostasis

2. Upright 45° Position

3. Correction of Anemia preferably with packed RBCs, and hypoxemia with oxygen.

4. Fluid Restriction (<120 cc/kg/day) and diuresis. Furosemide is the diuretic of choice in doses of 1 mg/kg per dose parenterally (total of 2 mg/kg) or 2 mg/kg per dose orally every six hours.

5. Digitalization (See below)

6. Inotropic Agents

    a. Isoproterenol, 0.1 to 0.2 μg/kg/min IV.

    b. Dopamine, 5 to 10 μg/kg/min IV.

7. Sedation with Assisted Ventilation can be used in the acute postoperative period of patients undergoing cardiac surgery.

8. Systemic Vasodilators are reserved for severe congestive heart failure unresponsive to traditional therapy. Such failure is usually manifested by decreased urine output, weight gain, poorly perfused extremities, alteration in levels of consciousness, or cardiogenic shock. Monitoring of arterial and filling pressure is required.

    a. Parenteral agent—nitroprusside, 1 to 8 μg/kg/min. The drug is contraindicated in liver and renal disease. Side effects of cyanide toxicity at thiocyanate levels of 0.5 to 1.0 mg/ml have been reported, with symptoms including nausea, fatigue, and anorexia.

b. Oral agent—prazosin hydrochloride, 25 µg/kg per dose every six hours.

9. Surgery

D. DIGITALIS

1. Digitalis has limited value in the newborn because of the inherent limited ability to increase stroke volume in response to load. Patients should be selected carefully.

   a. Individualize the digitalis dose. The usual total oral dose requirement is as follows:
      i. Premature infant, 0.04 mg/kg.
      ii. Term to 2 years, 0.05 to 0.07 mg/kg.

   b. Initial digitalization: one half of the calculated total dose immediately, one fourth in eight hours, and one fourth in 16 hours.

   c. Parenteral dose is two thirds of the calculated oral dose.

   d. Maintenance dose is one fourth of the total divided into two doses per day.

2. Normal Clinical Response to Digitalis Therapy

   a. Clinical improvement—respiratory effort, pulses, peripheral perfusion, decrease in liver size, slowing of heart rate.

   b. Digitalis effects on ECG—decreased heart rate, increased PR interval, T waves and ST segment depressed, sinus arrhythmia.

3. Symptoms of Digitalis Toxicity

   a. GI tract symptoms.

   b. Bradycardia, supraventricular tachycardia, PVCs or ventricular tachycardia, atrial fibrillation with AV block, or sinus rhythm with second- or third-degree AV block.

4. Laboratory Findings in Toxicity

   a. Serum potassium level may be low.

   b. Elevated digitalis level (>2 ng/cc). Level should be drawn six to eight hours after the last digoxin dose. Although 90% of patients with toxic reactions to digitalis have elevated levels, some patients tolerate more than 2 ng/cc without toxic effect.

5. Treatment of Toxic Reaction

a. Discontinue digitalis administration or skip one or two doses.

b. Give potassium chloride, 10 mEq/dl. Administer by slow drip 0.5 mEq/kg/hr and provide ECG monitoring. Potassium chloride is *contraindicated* in complete heart block.

c. Phenytoin, 2 to 4 mg/kg over five minutes.

d. Simple bradycardia without arrhythmia *is not* an indication to discontinue digitalis administration.

18

Patent Ductus Arteriosus
in the Premature Newborn

A. DIAGNOSIS

1. Symptoms of heart failure or difficulty in respiratory management (usually CO_2 retention), fluid or feeding intolerance, apnea.

2. Active precordium, and high-pitched systolic ejection murmur at the upper left sternal border.

3. Bounding pulses with wide BP and rapid diastolic pressure decay.

4. Occasionally hepatomegaly.

B. DIAGNOSTIC TESTS

1. **ECG** may be normal or have evidence of CVH, RVH, or LAH.

2. **Chest X-ray Film** look for cardiomegaly and increased vascularity.

3. **Echocardiogram** M mode estimations of LA, LV dimensions, LA/Ao ratio.

4. **Systolic Time Intervals** Shortening of ejection time on the left side, consistent with ductal runoff.

5. **Doppler Echocardiograph Evaluation** of ductal left-to-right shunt.

C. TREATMENT OF THE SYMPTOMATIC PDA CAN BE MEDICAL OR SURGICAL

1. Fluid restriction, anticongestive therapy, and maintenance of a normal hemoglobin level should be tried first.

2. If there is no response, indomethacin can be tried if there are no clinical or laboratory findings suggesting renal failure, hepatic failure, GI tract bleeding, thrombocytopenia, or necrotizing enterocolitis.

   a. Serum creatinine level should be less than 1.5 mg/dl, platelets count greater than 80,000/cu mm, and urine output normal.

   b. Indomethacin is given at a dose of 0.2 mg/kg per dose usually through a nasogastric tube. Intravenous indomethacin is not yet generally available, but is used in several centers.

   c. Indomethacin administration 0.1 mg/kg can be repeated up to three times at 12- to 24-hour intervals if urine output is adequate.

   d. If there is no initial response (with the above regimen), a subsequent response is unlikely.

3. Surgical closure of PDA is a safe alternative in cases where indomethacin therapy fails or is contraindicated.

19

Electrocardiography

A. NORMAL NEONATAL ECG INTERPRETATION

1. P Waves

a. P waves are normally upright in I, II, and AVF. Inverted P waves may indicate an ectopic atrial rhythm or dextrocardia.

b. Peaked P waves greater than 2.5 mm may be found in normal newborns and do not always indicate right atrial enlargement.

c. Broad notched P waves seen in left atrial enlargement is very rarely seen in the newborn.

2. PR Interval

a. PR interval should never exceed 0.11 seconds.

b. Prolonged PR interval is seen in primary AV conduction defects, endocardial cushion defects, digitalis effect, and bradycardia.

3. QRS

a. Duration: less than 0.09 seconds.

b. For frontal axis and amplitude, see Table 19–1.

4. QTc Corrected QT Interval

a. $QTc = QT\ interval/\sqrt{R - R\ interval}$ should not exceed 0.42 seconds.

b. Prolonged QTc is seen in hypocalcemia, hypokalemia, quinidine effect, metabolic derangements, and inherited (associated with arrhythmias, and, in some cases, deafness).

5. T Wave

a. Birth to five days—normally upright V_1-V_4, inverted V_5, V_6.

TABLE 19–1.—NORMAL NEONATAL ELECTROCARDIOGRAPHIC VALUES*

AGE (DAYS)	HEART RATE, (BEATS PER MINUTE) RANGE	FRONTAL QRS AXIS (DEGREES)		QRS AMPLITUDES CHEST LEADS (MILLIMETERS)					
				RIGHT (V₁, V₂) (RANGE)		LEFT (V₅, V₆) (RANGE)			
		MEAN	RANGE	R	S	R		S	
0–1	100–200	135	60–180	4.3–21	1.1–19.1	3.2–16.6		2.4–18.5	
1–7	100–180	125	80–160	3.3–18.7	0.0–15.0	3.8–24.2		2.8–16.3	
8–30	120–180	110	60–160	3.3–18.7	0.0–15.0	3.8–24.6		2.8–16.3	

*Adapted from Moss A.J., Adams F.H., Emmanouilides G.C. (eds): *Heart Disease in Infants, Children, and Adolescents*, ed 2. Baltimore, Williams & Wilkins Co., 1977, pp. 32–40.

   b. Five days to 30 days—normally inverted V_1-V_4, and upright V_5, V_6.

   c. Normal maximum T-wave amplitude: V_5 (95th percentile) 6 mm.

   d. T wave peaked in hyperkalemia: V_6 (95th percentile) 5 mm.

6. **Ventricular Hypertrophy**   Neonatal ECG is normally characterized by right ventricular dominance.

   a. Right ventricular hypertrophy is suggested by the following:
      i. R-wave amplitude in right precordial leads in excess of normal (see Table 19–1), or S-wave amplitude in left precordial leads in excess of normal.
      ii. Upright T waves in V_1, V_2 beyond five days or Q wave in right precordial leads.

   b. Left ventricular hypertrophy is suggested by the following:
      i. R-wave amplitude in left precordial leads in excess of normal, or S-wave amplitude in right precordial leads in excess of normal.
      ii. T-wave inversion in left precordial leads beyond five days or deep Q wave in left precordial leads, V_5, V_6, or large amplitude in limb leads (suggestive).

B. CONDUCTION DISORDERS

1. Atrioventricular Node (AV) Block

   a. First-degree AV block—PR interval greater than 0.12 seconds.

   b. Second-degree AV block.
      i. Type I (Wenckebach): Progressive lengthening of the PR interval until there is blocked AV node conduction and a dropped beat. Rhythm usually occurs with periodicity.
      ii. Type II: Dropped beats at regular intervals, may be 2:1 or 3:1 block.

   c. Complete AV block: No conducted atrial impulses. Atrial rate is greater than ventricular rate and ventricular rhythm is either junctional or idioventricular.

2. Bundle-Branch Block   Unusual in newborns.

   a. Complete left bundle-branch block.
      i. QRS duration greater than 0.10 seconds.
      ii. Broad monophasic R wave in lead I, and a wide S in V_1 and V_2.

iii. Left axis deviation.

b. Complete right bundle-branch block.
   i. QRS duration greater than 0.10 seconds.
   ii. An rSR' or rSR' complex in the right precordial leads.
   iii. Broad S wave in leads I, V_5, V_6.
   iv. Right axis deviation (suggestive).

C. RHYTHM DISTURBANCES

1. Premature Contractions

a. Premature atrial contractions (PACs) are very common in healthy newborns. Early P wave may be conducted or blocked. Conducted beats may be aberrant.

b. Premature junctional contractions are marked by early QRS with either inverted, absent, or retrograde P wave. Again, these are found commonly in healthy newborns.

c. Premature ventricular contractions are marked by broad complex QRS occurring before the expected atrial beat. They may be unifocal or multifocal (variable QRS morphology). Beats are usually followed by compensatory pause (which is twice the underlying RR interval).

2. Bradyarrhythmia   Slow heart rate

a. Sinus arrhythmia—normal P waves but P-P interval varies, usually with respiration, i.e., sinus rate increases during inspiration and decreases with expiration. This is often a normal finding.

b. Sinus bradycardia—normal P waves, but rate is less than expected for age. May be caused by both cardiac and extracardiac disorders.

c. Sinus node block and arrest. Very rarely seen in newborns. Long pause from dropped atrial beats.

3. Tachyarrhythmias   The tachyarrhythmias that require therapy are as follows:

a. Supraventricular—narrow QRS. This includes the following:
   i. Paroxysmal SVT—if symptomatic with heart failure or shock, then cardioversion with 1 watt-sec per pound then followed by prophylactic digoxin. If asymptomatic, perform vagal maneuvers or diving reflex and then digitalization.
   ii. Atrial flutter and fibrillation—cardioversion if symptomatic. Otherwise use digoxin and quinidine.

b. Ventricular
  i. Ventricular tachycardia—must first be differentiated from SVT with aberrancy. Ventricular tachycardia is supported by the presence of fusion beats, capture beats, and AV dissociation. If cardiac output is good, give a lidocaine bolus, 1 mg/kg. If successful, follow by lidocaine drip, 20 to 50 μg/kg/min. If the patient is symptomatic use cardioversion 1 watt-sec/lb followed by lidocaine drip.
  ii. Ventricular fibrillation—life threatening and treated by defibrillation 1 to 2 watt-sec/lb.

20

Echocardiography

A. M-MODE ECHOCARDIOGRAPHY IN THE NEWBORN

The m-mode echocardiogram can be used in the following ways:

1. Definition of Cardiac Anatomy

a. Identification of the four chambers and valves.

b. Establishing the relationship of the great arteries.

c. Used in conjunction with contrast echocardiography to elucidate intracardiac shunts.

2. Determination of Cardiac Chamber Size
Normal values for newborns are found in Table 20–1.

a. Left atrial diameter (LAD) size in infants with patent ductus arteriosus (PDA). Both the absolute LAD and LA/Ao ratio have been used to evaluate significance of left-to-right shunt: an La/Ao ratio greater than 1.2 is thought to be consistent with significant shunt.

b. Aortic root diameter is helpful in the diagnosis of aortic atresia and hypoplastic left heart syndrome.

c. Left ventricular end diastolic dimension (LVED) in LV volume loads, e.g., PDA or hydrops fetalis and condition of myocardial dysfunction, e.g., asphyxial cardiomyopathy.

d. Left ventricular posterior wall (LVPW) and interventricular septal thickness (IVS) in infants with LV outflow obstruction, e.g., congenital aortic stenosis, hypertrophic cardiomyopathy of infant of diabetic mother.

3. Cardiac Function
Left ventricular contractility as determined by shortening fraction percentage (SF%):
$$SF\% = (LVED - LVES)/LVED \times 100$$
The normal range is 27% to 40%.

TABLE 20–1.—NORMAL ECHOCARDIOGRAPHIC VALUES
FOR THE NEWBORN*

WEIGHT (KG)	LAD (CM)	AORTIC ROOT (CM)	LVED (CM)	RV (CM)	IVS (MM)	LVPW (MM)
<2.0	0.5–1.1	>0.5	0.9–1.6	. . .	. . .	. . .
2.0–4.9	0.6–1.3	0.7–1.2	1.2–2.4	0.6–1.5	1.8–4.5	1.6–4.6

*LAD indicates left atrial diameter; LVED, left ventricular end diastolic diameter; RV, right ventricular diameter; IVS, interventricular septal thickness; LVPW, LV posterior wall thickness.

4. **Systolic Time Intervals (STIs)** consist of pre-ejection period (PEP), ejection time (ET), and the PEP/ET ratio for right and left ventricle.

   a. LVSTI—useful in evaluating LV function. The LVPEP/LVET ratio is elevated in myocardial dysfunction (normal, 0.31 ∓ 0.05).

   b. RVSTI—useful in the evaluation of pulmonary resistance and pressures. The RVPEP/RVET ratio is elevated in pulmonary hypertension, i.e., persistent fetal circulation (normal ratios: less than five days, 0.26 to 0.35; greater than five days, 0.21 to 0.32).

B. 2-D ECHOCARDIOGRAPHY

Five 2-D planes are used to image the heart in the newborn.

1. **Parasternal Long-Axis View** is useful for evaluation of the LV, aortic and mitral valves, and certain types of VSDs, particularly in Fallot's tetralogy, truncus arteriosus, and double outlet right ventricle.

2. **Parasternal Short-Axis Views** are used to visualize the LV cavity, IVS, LVPW, and mitral valve or at a higher level the aortic and pulmonary valves and branch pulmonary arteries. This latter view is particularly helpful in the diagnosis of transposition of the great vessels.

3. **Apical Four-Chamber View** can be used to image simultaneously all four chambers and the two AV valves. Atrio-

ventricular valve disease, certain types of VSDs, and abnormalities of pulmonary venous return can be detected.

4. **Subcostal Views** are best for identifying atrial septal defects, locating and determining the size of VSDs, and assessing the right and left ventricular outflow tracts.

5. **Suprasternal View** is used primarily to evaluate the aortic arch and branch pulmonary arteries.

21

Neonatal Hypertension

A. DEFINITION

	Premature	Full-term	6-Weeks
Systolic BP	>80 mm Hg	>90 mm Hg	>115 mm Hg
Diastolic BP	>50 mm Hg	>60 mm Hg	. . .

B. ETIOLOGY

1. **Vascular Causes** include renal artery thrombosis, coarctation of the aorta, renal artery stenosis, and hypoplastic aorta.

2. **Renal Causes** include renal dysplasia, renal hypoplasia, obstructive uropathy, infantile polycystic disease, renal insufficiency, renal tumors, and nephrocalcinosis.

3. **Other Causes** include increased intracranial pressure, fluid and electrolyte overload, occular phenylephrine, neural crest tumor, adrenogenital syndrome, Cushing's disease (including iatrogenic), following correction of omphalocele, seizure, theophylline, and pneumothorax.

C. SIGNS AND SYMPTOMS

1. **Cardiorespiratory** Tachypnea, cyanosis, cardiomegaly.

2. **Neurological** Lethargy, tremors, seizures, hemiparesis, hypertonicity, and floppiness.

3. **Other** Nephromegaly, peripheral vascular occlusions.

4. **Asymptomatic**

D. EVALUATION

1. Abdominal ultrasound, IVP, peripheral plasma renin, serum creatinine, and BUN.

2. If there has been no use of an umbilical artery catheter:

   a. Rule out coarctation, corticosteroids or sympathomimetic drugs, increased intracranial pressure, or fluid and electrolyte overload.

   b. Blood pressure, upper and lower extremities, 24-hour urinary catecholamine, 17-hydroxysteroid, and 17-ketosteroid levels.

3. If renal artery thrombosis is suspected and an umbilical artery catheter is present, abdominal aortography or selective renal angiography should be done.

4. If the umbilical artery catheter has been withdrawn, ^{123}I or ^{131}I iodohippurate sodium renal scan, preferably with computer processing, is indicated: angiography should be done if the result of the scan is nondiagnostic.

E. MANAGEMENT

1. If possible, correct the underlying condition (GI tract obstruction, drugs, fluid overload) (Table 21–1).

2. Treat mild hypertension with diuretics and more severe hypertension with diuretics and hydralazine, beginning with 1 mg/kg/day and increasing the dosage up to 8 mg/kg/day. If the response is inadequate, add propranolol, beginning at 0.5 mg/kg/day and increasing to 3 mg/kg/day. If the response is still inadequate, add captopril, beginning at 0.05 mg/kg per dose and increasing *gradually* to 1.5 mg/kg per dose given every six to eight hours. Captopril is contraindicated with bilateral renal hypoperfusion or unilateral hypoperfusion in a solitary kidney (Table 21-1).

TABLE 21–1.—AGENTS USED
IN THE MANAGEMENT OF
NEONATAL HYPERTENSION

AGENT	RANGE (MG/KG/24 HR)
Chlorothiazide	20–50 mg/kg, orally
Furosemide	1–4 mg/kg IV, orally
Hydralazine	1–8 mg/kg IV, orally
Diazoxide	3–5 mg/kg/dose IV
Propranolol	0.5–3.0 mg/kg, orally
Nitroprusside	1.0–5 μg/kg/min IV
Captopril	0.05–1.5 mg/kg/dose

3. Life-threatening hypertension may be treated with diazoxide, 3 to 5 mg/kg/dose (which may cause severe hyperglycemia) or nitroprusside, 1.0–5.0 μg/kg/min. Blood pressure should be brought down gradually, not precipitously.

4. Consider nephrectomy if hypertension is caused by renal artery thrombosis and is not responding to maximal drug therapy.

22

Acute Renal Failure in Neonates

A. ETIOLOGY OF ACUTE RENAL FAILURE
(Table 22-1)

1. **Prerenal Causes** include asphyxia neonatorum, dehydration, congestive heart failure, or hypotension that may occur secondary to septic or cardiogenic shock, hemorrhage, or cardiac surgery.

2. **Renal Causes** include congenital abnormalities (cystic dysplasia, hypoplasia, agenesis, or polycystic kidneys), inflammatory or vascular (cortical necrosis, arterial thrombosis, or disseminated intravascular coagulation). An additional renal cause is acute tubular necrosis, which may occur secondary to perinatal asphyxia, dehydration, shock, or nephrotoxins, such as aminoglycosides.

3. **Postrenal Causes** include neurogenic bladder as well as obstruction that may occur secondary to posterior urethral valves, imperforate prepuce, urethral stricture or diverticulum, ureteropelvic or ureterovesical obstruction, or extrinsic tumors compressing bladder outlet.

B. DIAGNOSIS

1. **Oliguria**

a. Urinary output less than 1 ml/kg/hr

b. Confirm with catheterization

c. Assess the state of hydration. If patient is not clinically overhydrated, give isotonic saline, 20 ml/kg. If no response, give mannitol, 0.5 to 1.0 gm/kg. If no response, give furosemide, 1 to 4 mg/kg. If there is still no response, the patient is normovolemic and normotensive, and obstruction has been ruled out, treat the patient as having intrinsic renal failure.

2. **Elevated BUN** (>15 mg/dl) or elevated serum creatinine levels (>0.7 mg/dl) (not applicable during the first week of life), or a delayed postpartum decline in the serum creatinine value.

3. **Renal vs. Prerenal Failure** is illustrated in Table 22–2.

4. **Exclude Obstruction** based on clinical evaluation and, where necessary, perform abdominal ultrasound, renal scintography, or IV pyelography.

C. MANAGEMENT

1. **Give Insensible Water Loss** (full-term, 30 ml/kg; premature, 50 to 80 ml/kg) plus urinary output. Any deficit or ongoing losses such as nasogastric drainage or diarrhea should be replaced. Avoid overhydration, and weigh infant three times daily.

2. **No Sodium or Potassium** should be provided except to replace deficit or ongoing losses. Potassium repletion should be done carefully to avoid hyperkalemia. Hyponatremia is usually due to volume overload, not to sodium depletion.

3. **Significant Acidosis** should be corrected with sodium bicarbonate therapy to maintain a pH greater than 7.25.

4. **Hyperkalemia** may be treated with the following:

a. 10% calcium gluconate, 0.5 to 1.0 ml/kg given slowly IV.

b. Sodium bicarbonate, 2 mEq/kg, IV; glucose, 0.5 to 1.0 gm/kg, IV.

c. Intravenous insulin, one-quarter unit per gram of infused glucose.

d. Sodium polystyrene sulfonate, 1 gm/kg given orally or as a rectal enema.

e. Resistant hyperkalemia or acidosis should be treated with dialysis.

5. **Hyperphosphatemia** should be corrected with aluminum hydroxide gel, 2 to 5 cc/60 oz of oral intake and low-phosphate formulas PM 60/40 or SMA.

TABLE 22-1.—NORMAL RENAL FUNCTION IN THE NEONATE

	PREMATURE (<32 WK)	FULL-TERM	TWO WEEKS	TWO MONTHS
Glomerular filtration rate (ml/min/1.73 m)	10 ± 2	20 ± 5	40 ± 10	70 ± 10
Renal blood flow, ml/min	50 ± 10	85 ± 15	140 ± 20	240 ± 30
Maximum concentrating ability, (mOsm/L)	>600	>800	>1,000	>1,200
Excreted fraction of filtered sodium, %	3–8	<1	<1	<1

TABLE 22–2.—RENAL VS. PRERENAL FAILURE
IN NEWBORNS

	PRERENAL	RENAL
Urine osmolality, mOsm/kg of H_2O	>400	<400
Fractional excretion of sodium		
$U_{Na} \times S_{cr} \times 100/s_{Na} \times U_{cr}$	<3%*	>3%*
Renal Failure Index		
$U_{Na} \times S_{Cr}/U_{Cr} \times S_{Na}$	<3	>3

U_{Na} indicates urine sodium concentration; S_{Cr}, serum creatinine concentration; U_{Cr}, urine creatinine concentration; S_{Na}, serum sodium concentration.

*In infants at greater than 32 weeks of gestation.

6. **Asymptomatic Hypocalcemia** due to hyperphosphatemia should not be corrected until the serum phosphorus level is normalized, since a normal serum calcium level in the presence of hyperphosphatemia can lead to serious metastatic calcification. If the patient is clinically symptomatic, correct slowly with 10% calcium gluconate, 0.5 to 1.0 ml/kg intravenously until symptoms disappear.

7. **Protein** may be restricted to 1.5 to 2.0 gm/kg/day.

8. **A High Caloric Intake** using Polycose®, Controlyte®, or medium-chain triglycerides should be encouraged to minimize protein catabolism and generation of phosphate, sulfate, and urea.

9. Monitor weight, electrolyte level, intake, output, and vital signs frequently, and tabulate on flow sheets.

10. Modify dosage of drugs excreted by the kidneys (e.g., aminoglycosides).

11. Consult the nephrology service.

23

Hematuria

A. CAUSES

1. Perinatal hypoxia

2. Congenital malformations

3. Obstructive uropathy

4. Cortical and medullary necrosis

5. Renal vein thrombosis

6. Renal artery thrombosis

7. Hemorrhagic disease

8. Trauma

9. Urinary tract infection

10. Neoplasm

11. Glomerulonephritis (rare)

12. Hyperosmolar infusions

13. Nephrocalcinosis

B. EVALUATION

1. History of Predisposing Factors

a. Perinatal asphyxia: cortical or medullary necrosis.

b. Umbilical artery catheter: renal artery thrombosis with hypertension.

c. Maternal diabetes: renal vein thrombosis.

d. Furosemide usage: nephrocalcinosis.

2. **Abdominal Mass**   Renal vein thrombosis, obstructive uropathy, congenital malformation, or a renal neoplasm.

3. **Urinalysis**

a. Red blood cell casts suggestive of glomerulonephritis.

b. White blood cells and bacteriuria suggestive of urinary tract infection (with or without urinary tract malformations). Urinary tract infection should be confirmed by urine culture.

c. Crystals suggest a renal calculus, e.g., urate or calcium nephropathy.

4. Evidence of prolonged bleeding may suggest a bleeding diathesis.

5. Studies may include the following:

a. Urine calcium/creatinine ratio

b. Suprapubic tap for urine culture.

c. Clotting studies if bleeding diathesis suspected.

d. Abdominal ultrasound if mass is felt or nephrocalcinosis is suspected.

e. Intravenous pyelography.

f. Voiding cystourethrography.

g. Iodohippurate sodium ^{123}I or TC-DTPA renal scan.

h. Renal angiography.

24

Diarrhea and Malabsorption

Watery diarrhea indicates osmotic, secretory, or motility disorder. Steatorrhea manifests as foul-smelling, bulky, oily, greasy, pale stools.

A. DIAGNOSTIC TESTS

1. Screening Tests

a. *Examine* the stools for appearance.

b. Weigh stools separate from urine.

c. Test for occult blood (e.g., using Hemocult® slide method).

d. Examine the stool for inflammatory cells using methylene blue or *Wright's stain*. If any WBCs are seen, this indicates colitis.

e. Measure stool pH with nitrazine paper (pH 4.5–7.5). A pH greater than 5.5 indicates carbohydrate malabsorption (Table 24–1).

f. Test the stool for reducing (lactose, glucose), and nonreducing substances (sucrose).
   i. Mix one part stool and two parts water.
   ii. Centrifuge.
   iii. Transfer 15 drops of supernatant to a test tube.
   iv. Add Clinitest® tablet to supernatant and read color changes as urine Clinitest® result.

2. Specific Tests for Watery Diarrhea

a. A positive result using the Hemocult® method indicates mucosal injury. Perform a stool culture, kidney-ureter-bladder test, and proctosigmoidoscopy.

b. White blood cells on Wright's stain indicates colitis. Perform a stool culture, proctosigmoidoscopy, rectal biopsy, and barium enema.

TABLE 24–1.—Carbohydrate Tolerance Test

Place the infant on formula free of malabsorbed carbohydrate or make NPO so stool Clinitests® are < 0.25 percent.

Nothing by mouth for four to six hours.

Give orally sucrose as 20% solution or lactose 10% solution at 2 gm/kg per dose or 1 gm/kg of glucose and 1 gm/kg of galactose.

Obtain 0, 30-, and 60-minute blood glucose levels. A rise of blood glucose > 20 mg/dl with lactose and > 40 mg/dl with sucrose or glucose/galactose indicates normal absorption (10% to 15% false-positive rate).

Test all stools with Clinitest® and pH for 24 hours after oral challenge. Diarrhea stool with Clinitest® > ¼ percent and/or < 5.5 indicates malabsorption of that carbohydrate.

3. Specific Tests for Steatorrhea

a. Sweat chloride test using pilocarpine iontophoresis method of Gibson and Cooke. Greater than 70 mEq/L indicates cystic fibrosis.

b. Seventy-two-hour fecal fat balance study.
   i. Give charcoal orally at beginning and end of 72 hours to mark beginning and completion of stool collection.
   ii. Quantitative dietary fat during the 72 hours providing at least 4 gm/kg/24 hr of fat in the diet.
   iii. Coefficient of fat absorption =

$$\frac{\text{72-hr dietary fat (gm)} - \text{72-hr fecal fat (gm)}}{\text{72 hr. dietary fat (gm)}} \times 100\%$$

$$< 85\% = \text{fat malabsorption}$$

c. Other tests: stool trypsin, small intestinal biopsy, pancreatic stimulation.

B. DEFINITIVE DIAGNOSIS CAN USUALLY BE MADE

C. TREATMENT PER DIAGNOSIS

1. Elimination Diet

a. Breast milk or soy milk for cow's milk allergy.

b. Breast milk or Nutramigen for cow's milk and soy milk allergy.

    c. Soy milk for lactase deficiency.

    d. Pregestimil for lactase and sucrase-isomaltase deficiency or pancreatic exocrine insufficiency.

    e. Hyperalimentation if all carbohydrates are malabsorbed or if there is severe secretory diarrhea (greater than 50-gm stool in 24 hours while nothing by mouth).

2. Treat infection with antibiotics.

3. Pancreatic enzymes for pancreatic enzyme deficiency.

4. MCT oil for bile salt deficiency or defects in fat transport.

5. Surgical correction of Hirschsprung's disease.

REFERENCES

1. Ament M.E.: Malabsorption syndromes in infancy and childhood. *J. Pediatr.* 81:685–697, 867–884, 1972.
2. Gall D.J., Hamilton M.R.: Chronic diarrhea in childhood. *Pediatr. Clin. North Am.* 21:1001–1017, 1974.

25

Gastrointestinal Tract Bleeding

Gastrointestinal tract bleeding in the neonate may occasionally be severe and treatment should be initiated promptly. To treat the bleeding appropriately, the bleeding site should be identified if possible. With current diagnostic techniques, 90% of bleeding sites can be identified (50% anus, rectum, colon, 30% small intestine, 10% above ligament of Treitz).

A. BLEEDING SITES

1. Upper GI tract

a. Stress (birth, cardiac disease, sepsis—antrum most common)

b. Drugs (steroids, indomethacin, salicylates, caffeine, tolazoline)

c. Esophagitis (gastroesophageal reflux, nasogastric tubes).

d. Coagulopathy

e. Other (duplication cysts, Mallory-Weiss tear, AV malformation, hemangioma, milk bezoar)

2. Small Bowel

3. Anus, Rectum, and Colon

a. Colitis (infection, cow's milk or soy protein allergy, Hirschsprung's disease)

b. Anal fissure

B. DIAGNOSTIC TESTS

1. Physical Examination

a. Hypotension, tachycardia, or both suggest at least 20% of blood volume lost.

b. Bruising or bleeding from other sites suggests coagulopathy.

c. Hepatosplenomegaly and jaundice suggest coagulopathy secondary to liver disease.

d. Abdominal distention and mass suggest duplication cyst, intussusception, or midgut volvulus.

e. Hemangioma or AV malformations on skin suggest similar lesions in GI tract.

f. Presence of nasogastric tube may implicate this as a source of mucosal injury.

2. **Aspiration of Nasogastric Secretion** may demonstrate upper GI tract bleeding site. However, if there is no blood in the nasogastric aspirate, this indicates that bleeding has ceased or that it is beyond the pylorus.

3. **Laboratory Tests** stool guaiac, KUB, PT, PTT, platelet count, hematocrit reading, hemoglobin values.

4. **Other Diagnostic Studies**

a. Proctosigmoidoscopy will identify most lower GI bleeding sites such as colitis or anal fissures. Rectal biopsy will show colitis when it may not be apparent on proctosigmoidoscopy and will rule out Hirschsprung's disease.

b. Upper endoscopy and colonscopy can now be performed on neonates with pediatric fiberoptic flexible scopes. More than 90% of bleeding sites can be identified with these instruments.

c. Barium enema is diagnostic test when KUB result suggests obstruction, Hirschsprung's disease, or intussusception. Intussusception in a neonate is usually associated with anatomic malformation such as duplication cyst.

d. If bleeding is massive then angiography or technetium 99m scan should be performed to identify sites. Angiography is better when the bleeding is greater than 0.5 ml/min, while the latter is more sensitive at less than 0.1 ml/min but less specific.

C. TREATMENT

1. Place appropriate arterial/venous lines to monitor BP and CVP.

2. Replace blood losses with blood or other volume expanders (e.g., fresh-frozen plasma, Ringer's lactate, or albumin) if blood is not available.

3. Control bleeding by correcting coagulopathy, discontinuing inappropriate drugs.

   a. Correct coagulopathy with fresh-frozen plasma, vitamin K, or platelet packs.

4. Lavage blood from stomach with saline at room temperature.

5. Antacids.

6. Antibiotics (colitis).

7. Necrotizing enterocolitis (NEC) should be treated by bowel rest (making the neonates NPO), antibiotics, and total parenteral nutrition.

8. Surgical intervention should be immediate for obstructive lesions such as midgut volvulus, intussusception, for toxic megacolon due to Hirschsprung's disease, and for Meckel's diverticulum. If bleeding continues with greater than 85 cc/kg/24 hr of blood loss, surgical exploration for control of bleeding is advised.

REFERENCES

1. Cox K.L., Ament M.G.: Upper gastrointestinal bleeding in children and adolescents. *Pediatrics* 63:408–413, 1979.
2. Sherman N.J., Clatsworthy H.W. Jr.: Gastrointestinal bleeding in neonates: A study of 94 cases. *Surgery* 62:614, 1967.

26

Common Surgical Problems

A. NECROTIZING ENTEROCOLITIS

1. **Pathophysiological Findings** include an ischemic lesion of the intestine, with bacterial infection playing a contributory role. Feeding insults the gut by placing further demands on an already compromised situation.

2. **Clinical Presentation and Diagnosis**

   a. Mild to fulminant, presents anytime in first six weeks of life.

   b. More common in premature infants.

   c. The earliest sign is often intolerance of feedings (gastric residuals).

   d. Diagnosis: pneumatosis intestinalis, portal air, pneumoperitoneum on KUB test.

3. **Management**

   a. Stop feedings if distention is present.

   b. Place nasogastric tube for GI decompression.

   c. Administer systemic antibiotics.

   d. Perform frequent abdominal x-rays. Technetium Tc 99m pyrophosphate scan should be considered.

   e. Begin TPN when stable.

   f. Surgery is indicated for perforation, progressive deterioration, or late stricture.

B. DIAPHRAGMATIC HERNIA

1. **Pathophysiological Findings** Defects (Bochdalek's hernia in posterior lateral diaphragm) allow abdominal contents to fill the chest and compromise lung development *bilaterally*.

Ninety percent of diaphragmatic hernias occur on the left. Pulmonary hypertension usually occurs as well.

2. Clinical Presentation and Diagnosis

a. Respiratory distress, decreased breath sounds on the affected side, shift of heart sounds to the opposite side, and scaphoid abdomen are classic findings.

b. Chest x-ray film reveals opacity or bowel in the chest.

3. Management

a. Ventilation by endotracheal tube. (Mask ventilation is contraindicated due to inflation of the gut.)

b. Pulmonary vasodilators, if indicated.

c. Operative repair.

C. INTESTINAL OBSTRUCTION

1. Pathophysiological Findings   Intrauterine vascular accident, cystic fibrosis, meconium ileus, Hirschsprung's disease, error in rotation or fixation.

2. Clinical Presentation and Diagnosis

a. Bilious vomiting. Cause must be established without delay.

b. Failure of passage of meconium within 24 hours in a baby being fed or within 48 hours in a baby being kept NPO is abnormal.

c. Abdominal distention, visible intestinal loops, or obvious peritonitis.

d. Rectal examination should not be performed until all x-ray examinations are completed.

3. Management

a. Nasogastric suction.

b. Chest or abdominal x-ray films should include the pelvis.

c. Meconium obstruction is diagnosed and usually treated by contrast enema with hypertonic water-soluble agents.

d. Decompressive colostomy is the treatment of Hirschsprung's disease.

D. ABDOMINAL WALL DEFECT

1. **Pathophysiological Findings** Protrusion of the midgut, its return, rotation, fixation, and subsequent closure of the abdominal wall occurring in the first trimester before complete formation of the abdominal wall.

2. **Types**

   a. Omphalocele is a defect with the abdominal contents covered by peritoneum and amnion.

   b. In gastroschisis, the peritoneal/amnion membrane is absent. The cord is usually to the left of the defect.

3. **Extrophy,** a rare anomaly, occurs with lower abdominal embryogenetic defects.

4. **Management**

   a. Infants with omphalocele or hernia of the cord with intact membrane should receive nasogastric suction. The sac should be kept moist with saline-soaked gauze and plastic wrap.

   b. The herniated bowel in gastroschisis, or ruptured omphalocele, can suffer vascular compromise if its blood supply is kinked over the edge of the defect. The baby should be turned on his side to avoid vascular embarrassment. A nasogastric tube should be placed. Saline-moist gauze and plastic wrap or a plastic bag should be used to keep the intestine moist. Evaporative losses are large and IV hydration is important. Antibiotics for systemic effect are given.

   c. Primary closure is the ideal procedure. Temporary prosthetic pouches are used to allow slow reduction of abdominal contents if primary closure is not possible. Antiseptic painting of intact omphalocele sac is used if operative closure is not performed.

E. IMPERFORATE ANUS

1. **Pathophysiological Findings** A spectrum of anomalies that can be classed as either low-type (intralevator) or high-type (supralevator) depending on the location of the terminus of the colon. Fistula to the vagina is common in all types of

imperforate anus in females. In males with high-type anomalies, fistula to the urinary tract (usually urethral) is common.

2. Clinical Presentation and Diagnosis

a. Diagnosis is not often a problem. Distinction between high- and low-type can be difficult. X-rays can be helpful. Serial examination watching for meconium passing through a fistula or in the urine is important.

b. An adequate-sized nasogastric tube should be passed for decompression as well as to rule out esophageal atresia (associated in 10% of cases).

3. Management

a. Local peritoneal procedures are performed in low-type imperforate anus and include dilation, "cut-back," anoplasty, or anal transposition.

b. High-type anomalies are treated with colostomy initially. Pull-through procedures are performed after six months or later.

F. TRACHEOESOPHAGEAL FISTULA

1. Clinical Presentation and Diagnosis

a. Maternal polyhydramnios, excess oral secretions, inability to feed, gagging.

b. Lateral and AP x-ray of the thoraco-cervical region and abdomen usually will suffice for diagnosis, showing blind pouch and air in GI tract.

c. Isolated esophageal atresia or tracheoesophageal fistula (TEF) have absence of gas in GI tract.

2. Principals of Preoperative Management

a. Minimal disturbance of infant to prevent reflux and aspiration of acid gastric secretions.

b. Keep infant inclined in a 60°, head-up prone position.

c. Avoid manipulative procedures if possible.

3. Usual Operative Procedure

a. Transection of TEF and end-to-end anastomosis of proximal and distal esophagus.

b. If the gap between esophageal segments is too large for

primary anastomosis, the fistula is ligated and delayed anastomosis follows stretching of the upper segment by serial bougienage.

4. Principles of Postoperative Management

a. If a primary anastomosis can be made, NPO with TPN for one to two weeks.

b. If the primary anastomosis cannot be made, gastrostomy feeds are started around the third postoperative day.

27

Hemostatic Disorders

A. NORMAL VALUES

Normal values for routine coagulation tests are considerably different for preterm infants weighing less than 1,500 gm than for larger newborns (Table 27–1).

B. DIAGNOSIS

Any clinically apparent hemostatis problem requires a series of initial laboratory tests. The diagnostic approach is summarized as follows:

 a. Initially obtain the following:
 Platelet count
 Partial thromboplastin time (PTT)
 Prothrombin time (PT)

TABLE 27–1.—NORMAL VALUES FOR TERM AND PRETERM INFANTS*

AGE	ACTIVATED PTT (SEC)	PT (SEC)	TT (SEC)
Child	30–40	10–12	10–15
Full-term			
(cord)	70	12–17	10–20
(48 hrs)	60	12–20	10–16
Preterm (31 weeks)			
(cord)	105	15–22	15–20
(48 weeks)	75	15–22	15–20

*Platelet count range for all ages is 180,000 to 300,000/cu mm. Clottable fibrinogen level for all ages is 150 to 250 mg/dl.
 PTT indicates partial thromboplastin time; PT, prothrombin time; TT, thrombin time.

Thrombin (TT)
Clottable fibrinogen (I_C)

    b. If all values are normal, perform bleeding time and urea solubility tests.
      i. If bleeding time is prolonged, this suggests platelet dysfunction or von Willebrand's disorder.
      ii. If urea solubility is abnormal, this suggests factor XIII deficiency.

    c. If panel "a" is abnormal, characterize the pattern of abnormality, e.g., *decreased platelet count* with normal PTT, PT, TT, I_C, or normal platelet count with *prolonged PTT,* normal PT, TT I_C, etc. (Table 27–2). Order assays to delineate defect.

C. INHERITED DEFECTS

1. Platelet-Vessel Wall Disorders

    a. Von Willebrand's disorder is an autosomally inherited disorder characterized by a prolonged bleeding time and variable abnormalities of the factor VIII molecule. Clinical hemorrhage is unusual in the neonate except in patients with the homozygous form. The laboratory work-up includes a bleeding time and factor VIII molecule assessment (factor VIII coagulant, factor VIII mulitimer assay) of both parents and patient.

    b. Severe platelet function defects are rare. Conditions to be considered are Glanzmann's thrombasthenia, Bernard-Soulier syndrome (platelet membrane glycoprotein defects), prostaglandin synthesis disorders (enzyme defects), and granulocyte storage pool disorders.

2. Procoagulant Disorders

    a. The hemophilias, factor VIII, IX, or XI are characterized, in the severe and moderate form, by a prolonged PTT and otherwise normal hemostatic screening test results. Factor VIII and IX defects are inherited as sex-linked recessive traits, whereas factor XI is autosomally inherited with a high frequency to Ashkenazi Jews.

    b. Isolated deficiencies of other factors are very rare in comparison with the hemophilias.

TABLE 27–2.—Patterns of Laboratory Screening Tests*

	A	B	C	D	E	F
Platelet count	low	nl	nl	nl	nl	nl
PTT	nl	prolonged†	nl	nl	nl	prolonged†
PT	nl	nl	prolonged†	nl	nl	prolonged†
TT	nl	nl	nl	prolonged†	nl	nl
I_c	nl	nl	nl	nl	low	nl

*Column headings indicate the following test procedures:

A. Work-up for thrombocytopenia includes platelet sizing, review of peripheral blood smear, maternal platelet count, sizing and platelet-associated IgG antibody, and consideration of bone marrow aspirate.

B. Work-up includes assay for factors VIII, IX, XI.

C. Work-up includes assay for factors X, V, II.

D. Work-up includes assay for fibrin(ogen) degradation products.

E. Work-up includes factor VII assay in addition to other liver vitamin K–dependent factor assays.

F. Work-up includes administration of vitamin K_1 followed by repeated PT and PTT in four hours.

If still abnormal, assay for factors V, VII, X, and fibrinogen.

PTT indicates partial thromboplastin time; PT, prothrombin time; TT, thrombin time; I_C, clottable fibrinogen; nl, normal.

†A prolonged PTT, PT, or TT should initially be assessed as to presence of inhibitor in system by performing an in vitro mixing experiment of 1:1 mixture of patients plasma and normal pooled plasma with repeat of screening test. If the initially prolonged test fails to correct *completely* to the normal range, the presence of an inhibitor may be suspected, e.g., heparin, degradation products, lupus anticoagulant, etc.

D. ACQUIRED DEFECTS

1. Platelet-Vessel Wall Disorders

a. The most common defect of the hemostatic system is an acquired disorder of platelet function secondary to the effects of drugs administered either to the mother or to the neonate. Clinical bleeding is uncommon, but may add to the patient's morbidity if hemorrhage occurs for some other reason, e.g., thrombocytopenia.

2. Procoagulant Disorders

a. Procoagulant factor defects may occur as a result of vitamin K deficiency, secondary to inadequate supply of vitamin K, or as a result of medications that interfere with vitamin K availability (antibiotics) or that block vitamin K action (anticonvulsants).

b. The most common procoagulant defect observed relates to the sick neonate in whom an exaggerated hypocoagulable state develops due to a combination of intravascular coagulation and decreased ability to produce adequate amounts of procoagulant proteins. The spectrum of laboratory abnormalities varies from all coagulation tests being prolonged secondary to a decreased fibrinogen level (<80 mg/dl), to only one of the tests being prolonged (PTT, PT, TT). The etiology of this spectrum of abnormalities usually includes infection, liver disease, hypoxia, or any combination of these problems.

E. TREATMENT

1. Once the laboratory test results have been obtained, treatment should be instituted rapidly in the infant with clinical bleeding. If the platelet count is below 50,000/cu mm, consideration of platelet transfusion should be undertaken. A single unit of platelets administered to the neonate will usually increase the platelet count by 40,000 to 50,000/cu mm. In addition, each platelet pack has 35 to 50 ml of fresh plasma and, therefore, if the procoagulant tests are prolonged, partial correction of this defect can be accomplished simultaneously (10 m/kg of fresh plasma will increase any single procoagulant factor level by 10% to 15%).

2. Hypofibrinogenemia can best be corrected by infusion of cryoprecipitate. One unit or bag of cryoprecipitate (average vol-

ume, 10 to 15 ml) per kilogram of body weight will increase the fibrinogen level by 50 mg/dl and provide more than adequate levels of fibrinogen for hemostatis. Cryoprecipitate also contains fibronectin and factor XIII.

3. Fresh-frozen plasma can be used at dosages of 10 ml/kg to partially correct most procoagulant deficiencies until such time that a definitive diagnosis is established, whereupon specific factor replacement therapy can be given, e.g., hemophilia A or factor VIII replacement therapy.

4. The frequency of repeated transfusions of any given material depends on close monitoring of hemostatis measurements after transfusion and knowledge of the half-life of each deficient component.

F. THROMBOTIC DISORDERS

Defects of the hemostatic system leading to or perpetuating thrombosis in the neonate include consideration of antithrombin III, protein C, and prostacyclin deficiency states. At present, no laboratory screening tests are available for these deficiencies, but rather specific assessment is required, i.e., ATIII assay.

REFERENCES

1. Oski F.A., Naiman J.L.: *Hematologic Problems in the Newborn,* ed 3. Philadelphia, W.B. Saunders Co., 1982.
2. Hathaway W.E., Bonnar J.: *Perinatal Coagulation.* New York, Grune & Stratton, 1978.

28

Anemia

A. Anemia may be present at birth or develop postnatally following blood loss, hemolysis, or decreased red cell production. Normal values are shown in Table 28–1.

B. GENERAL APPROACH

Identify and correct the cause, replacing blood as needed.

1. The cause is usually obvious from the history or physical examination.

2. When the cause is not apparent:

   a. Review prenatal and perinatal history for evidence of uterine trauma, perinatal blood loss, or delivery problems.

   b. Obtain hematocrit and hemoglobin values (serial), reticulocyte count, and RBC smear for morphological findings.

   c. Consider Coombs' test on infant blood and Kleihauer-Betke test using maternal blood.

3. General Indications for Treatment Base decision on whether physiological or biochemical effect of anemia places the infant at risk.

   a. In oxygen-dependent patients with compromised oxygen-carrying capacity, it may be desirable to maintain a hematocrit reading above 35% to 40%, depending on energy expenditure.

   b. Infants requiring frequent blood sampling should receive packed RBC transfusions when about 10% of their blood volume has been removed.

   c. In convalescent babies transfusions will simply delay the normal physiologic anemia of the newborn and activation of erythropoiesis. Symptomatic infants should be treated.

TABLE 28-1.—NORMAL VALUES FOR FULL-TERM INFANTS*†

AGE	HEMOGLOBIN, (g/dl)	RBCs (10⁶ μL)	HEMATOCRIT (%)	MCV (μm3)	RETICULOCYTE COUNT (%)
Cord blood	14.6–19.6	5.4	56.6	106	3.2
Day 1	21.2 (18.2)	5.6 (4.7)	56.1	106 (115)	3.2
Day 7	19.6 (16.3)	5.3 (4.4)	52.7	101 (110)	0.5
Day 14	18.0 (14.5)	5.1 (4.1)	49.6	96 (106)	0.8
Day 21	16.6 (12.9)	4.9 (3.7)	46.6	93 (102)	0.6
Day 28	15.6 (10.9)	4.7 (3.2)	44.6	91 (100)	0.9

*( ) indicates values for low-birth-weight infants. RBCs indicates red blood cells; MCV, mean corpuscular volumes.

†From Stockman A.M., Oski F.: Normal hematocrit and MCV. *Am. J. Dis. Child.* 134:94, 1980. Used by permission.

Symptoms attributable to anemia are as follows:
  i. Weight gain falls off.
  ii. Decreased activity, feeding, and responsiveness.
  iii. Baseline heart rate increases more than 20 beats per minute.
  iv. Apneic episodes appear or increase in frequency.

4. **General Treatment** Give packed RBCs, 10 ml/kg (maximum, 15 m/kg) IV over a period of 30 to 60 minutes. This will usually raise the hemoglobin level 2 to 4 gm/dl.

5. **Specific Causes, Diagnosis, and Management**

   a. Fetal-maternal transfusion: Review maternal history for uterine trauma. Obtain Kleihauer-Betke acid elution test for fetal cells in mother's blood. Large transfusion could sensitize the mother to minor blood groups or require additional Rh(D) globulin if Rh incompatible.

   b. Identical twin-twin transfusion. Both twins may need adjustment of hematocrit.

   c. Obstetrical bleeding: abruption, placenta previa, torn umbilical cord, placental incision during cesarean section.
      i. The infant may have a normal hematocrit reading at birth and not show obvious shock despite substantial blood loss.
      ii. Measure central hematocrit on admission to the nursery and four hours later. Correct with volume if metabolic acidosis is present or if blood pressure is low.

   d. Internal hemorrhage: Covert serious bleeding may result from rupture of liver (most common) or spleen following difficult delivery. Shock, anemia, or both may be delayed with rupture of liver capsule, which temporarily tamponades subcapsular hemorrhage.

   e. Hemolysis may result from acute or chronic infection, isoimmune hemolytic disease, inherited defects in red cell membrane structure, or enzyme deficiencies. When severe, RBC morphological findings are often characteristic.
      i. Spherocytes: ABO incompatibility, hereditary spherocytosis.
      ii. Erythroblasts: Severe intrauterine hemolytic disease (usually Rh isoimmune disease).
      iii. Fragmented cells, burr cells: Infection DIC, metabolic disease.
      iv. RBC membrane defects (rare), elliptocytosis, stomatocytosis, etc.
      v. Microcytic, hypochromic: α-thalassemia.

f. Production defects: Suspect when newborn has severe anemia and reticulocytopenia.
  i. Usually due to infection or maternal drugs.
  ii. Aplastic anemias (e.g., Blackfan-Diamond syndrome) are rarely apparent in the first weeks of life.

g. Delayed-onset anemia
  i. Physiologic anemia of convalescing premature infant. Monitor hematocrit reading weekly or more frequently.
  ii. Vitamin E deficiency is characterized by normal blood smear, high reticulocyte count, high platelet count, frequently peripheral edema, and low plasma tocopherol level. Treat with vitamin E, 25 IU/day until plasma level vitamin E normalizes.

REFERENCES

1. Oski-Naiman: Major problems in clinical pediatrics, in *Hematologic Problems in the Newborn,* ed 2. Philadelphia, W.B. Saunders Co., 1982.
2. Lamzkowsky: Diagnosis of anemia in the neonatal period and during childhood, in chap, *Pediatric Hematology-Oncology.* McGraw-Hill, 1980, pp 3–41.

29

Polycythemia/Hyperviscosity

Hyperviscosity syndrome may be associated with a wide variety of signs and symptoms, immediate complications, and long-term sequelae. The main determinant of blood viscosity is the hematocrit reading. However, viscosity is also increased by any factor that decreases the deformability of blood. Because blood viscosity measurements are not generally available, the diagnosis is usually based on an elevated hematocrit reading (polycythemia).

A. INCIDENCE

Hyperviscosity syndrome occurs in about 2% to 5% of newborns, as well as in the following:

1. About 3% to 4% of AGA term infants.

2. About 8% LGA and SGA infants.

3. There is a higher occurrence in infants of diabetic mothers, in trisomies (13, 18, 21), and in cases of placental insufficiency, twin-twin transfusion, and placental transfusion at birth.

4. It is rare at less than 34 weeks' gestation.

B. CLINICAL FEATURES

1. **Polycythemia**   may occur with or without accompanying signs of symptoms.

2. **Neurological**   Lethargy, hypotonia or hypertonia, difficulty in arousing, irritability, tremulousness, poor sucking and feeding, vomiting.

3. **Physical**   Plethora, cyanosis when crying, tachypnea, heart failure, hepatomegaly, ileus, jaundice.

4. **Biochemical**   Hypoglycemia, hypocalcemia, hyperbilirubinemia.

5. **Roentgenographic**   Cardiomegaly, increased pulmonary vascular markings.

6. **Other**   Thrombocytopenia, abnormal EEG, ECG.

C. OUTCOME

1. Neonatal Complications

a. Congestive heart failure.

b. Infarction of peripheral appendages, brain, renal vein, gut (necrotizing enterocolitis).

c. Neonatal signs and symptoms will usually improve following partial exchange transfusion to reduce viscosity.

2. Long-Term Neurological or Developmental Sequelae

a. If the baby is asymptomatic in the nursery, it is not certain whether long-term complications occur.

b. If the baby is symptomatic in the nursery, subsequent difficulties may arise, particularly if polycythemia is accompanied by hypoglycemia.

c. Complications other than those resulting from major infarction include minimal neurological findings, e.g., mild deficits in speech, hearing, or coordination. Serious complications include spastic diplegia and mental retardation. It is uncertain whether long-term complications can be prevented in the neonatal period.

D. DIAGNOSIS

1. Diagnosis Is Complicated by the Following Relationships:

a. Hyperviscosity is defined arbitrarily as two standard deviations above the mean for a tested population.

b. Although hematocrit (Hct) is the principle determinant of viscosity, other factors such as acidosis, hypoxia, spherocytosis, etc., which decrease RBC deformability, may increase viscosity at a given hematocrit reading.

   c. Viscosity increases more rapidly with small increases in the hematocrit reading at higher hematocrit levels.

   d. Hematocrit in capillary blood obtained from heel stick (Hct_c), antecubital venous blood (Hct_v), and umbilical venous blood may differ. The Hct_c is particularly unreliable during the first four to six hours of life.

2. We Use the Following Approach for Diagnosing Polycythemia:

   a. An Hct_c should be performed on all plethoric or symptomatic babies at 4 to 6 hours of age.

   b. If the Hct_c is greater than or equal to 70%, a Hct_v should be drawn from an antecubital vein.

   c. If the Hct_c is greater than 65% *and* the infant is symptomatic, a Hct_v should also be drawn.

   d. If the Hct_v is greater than 65% the diagnosis of polycythemia is made.

E. CRITERIA FOR TREATMENT

1. Symptomatic Infants
If the Hct_v is greater than 65% and the infant has clinical features compatible with hyperviscosity syndrome, a partial exchange transfusion should be performed.

2. Asymptomatic Infants
Currently available evidence does not permit a recommendation regarding intervention in this group of infants. If the Hct_v is greater than 70%, the infant should be monitored carefully for neurological and biochemical abnormalities and treatment based on their appearance.

F. TREATMENT
Partial exchange transfusion to reduce Hct_v to about 55%.

1. Calculation of Blood Volume to Be Exchanged

   a. Assume blood volume of 80 to 90 cc/kg (may be higher if polycythemia is due to placental transfusion).

   b. Calculation:
$$\text{volume exchanged} = [\text{blood volume} \times (Hct - 55)]/Hct_v$$

2. Partial Exchange Transfusion
may be performed through a low umbilical vein catheter advanced 3 to 5 cm until

there is good blood return or through a low umbilical artery catheter.

3. **Obtain a Central Hematocrit Reading** before and after the exchange transfusion (before removing the catheter).

4. **Withdraw Blood**   in 10-ml aliquots and replace with an equal volume of plasmanate. Fresh-frozen plasma is more expensive and is not usually required for this procedure.

REFERENCES

1. Ramamurthy R.S., Brans V.W.: Neonatal polycythemia: I. Criteria for diagnosis and treatment. *Pediatrics* 68:168–174, 1981.
2. Black V.D., Lubchenco L.O., Luckey D.W., et al.: Developmental and neurologic sequelae of neonatal hyperviscosity syndrome. *Pediatrics* 69:426–431, 1982.

30

Jaundice

Evaluation of jaundice in newborns presents two distinct problems. First, unconjugated bilirubin can be toxic and cause irreversible neurological damage; second, jaundice may also be a sign of an underlying disease.

A. JAUNDICE MAY BE A POSTNATAL ADAPTIVE (PHYSIOLOGICAL) OR DISEASE PROCESS

1. Differentiating between physiological and pathological bilirubinemia in a given patient is based on statistical data, and by excluding alternative explanations of the jaundice. Presume a pathological cause if the serum bilirubin level is greater than 7, 9, or 11 mg/dl at 24, 48, or 72 hours of age, respectively.

2. In the premature infant, the bilirubin concentration may rise faster and reach maximum elevations on the fourth or fifth day of life as compared with the third day in term infants.

3. When the serum bilirubin concentration exceeds values that can be statistically assumed to result from physiological adaptation, *or* you choose to place the baby under phototherapy, then the cause of the jaundice *must* be investigated.

B. DIFFERENTIAL DIAGNOSIS OF UNCONJUGATED (INDIRECT) HYPERBILIRUBINEMIA

See Table 30–1

TABLE 30–1.—DIFFERENTIAL DIAGNOSIS OF UNCONJUGATED
HYPERBILIRUBINEMIA*

Hemolytic Disease
Isoimmune hemolytic disease
  RH incompatibility
  ABO incompatibility
  Minor blood group incompatibility

Inherited RBC metabolic disorders
  Glucose-6-phosphate dehydrogenase
    deficiency (sex linked)
  Pyruvate kinase deficiency

Disorders in RBC morphology
  Hereditary spherocytosis
  Infantile pyknocytosis

Infections
Bacterial sepsis
TORCH infections

Toxins
  Excess dose vitamin K

Metabolic Disorders
Galactosemia
Crigler-Najjar disease
Breast milk jaundice
Familial neonatal
  jaundice
  (Lucey-Driscoll
  syndrome)
Infants of diabetic
  mothers
Hypothyroidism

Other Causes
High intestinal obstruction
Enclosed hemorrhage
  (e.g.,
  cephalohematoma)
Swallowed maternal
  blood

*Causes of obstructive jaundice (elevated direct fraction) are not included in
this table. Elevated direct reading bilirubin may or may not be a feature of infection or erythroblastosis fetalis.

C. EVALUATION OF THE JAUNDICED INFANT

1. **History** (particularly positive family history of the following:
   hemolytic disease, Lucey-Driscoll syndrome, breast milk jaundice, or diabetes).

2. **Physical Examination** Prematurity, organomegaly, pro-
   truding tongue with umbilical hernia, poor feeding, large
   fontanelle, petechiae, bruising, obesity (infant of diabetic
   mother).

3. Laboratory

a. Serum bilirubin (direct/total)

b. Red blood cell smear
   i. Rh incompatibility—nucleated RBCs, erythroblasts
   ii. ABO incompatibility—microspherocytes
   iii. Sepsis, glucose-6-phosphate dehydrogenase deficiency—fragmented RBC
   iv. Pyknocytosis—pyknocytes

c. Blood type, Rh determination, and Coombs' test on mother and infant

d. Hematocrit or hemoglobin values

e. Other (persistent jaundice, other tests not diagnostic)
   i. Urine culture to rule out urinary tract infection
   ii. Urine Clinitest® (galactosemia)
   iii. Thyroxine (T$_4$) and thyroid-stimulating hormone (TSH)

4. Only after careful consideration has been given to serious disease can a diagnosis of "idiopathic hyperbilirubinemia" safely be assigned an infant.

D. EVALUATING RISK FOR KERNICTERUS

1. Monitor the bilirubin level to establish rate of rise and peak value.

a. Hemolytic disease—every four to six hours in first day until the rate of rise is established; then every six to eight hours until two sequential samples show decline.

b. Nonhemolytic jaundice—every eight to 12 hours in a baby whose bilirubin level is increasing, and every six to eight hours when bilirubin approaches the exchange level.

c. Bilirubin level declining or stable—every 12 to 24 hours or longer depending on the vulnerability of the patient.

2. Factors increasing the susceptibility of tissue to bilirubin toxicity include asphyxia, hypoglycemia, acidosis, chronic intrauterine asphyxia, and meningitis.

3. Bilirubin-albumin binding tests may improve the estimation of risk for encephalopathy.

a. We use both front-face fluorometry (Hematofluorometer) and free bilirubin determinations (apparent unbound bilirubin

TABLE 30–2.—ACCEPTABLE INDICATIONS FOR EXCHANGE TRANSFUSION
(INDIRECT BILIRUBIN, MG/DL)

BASIS	>2,500 GM	<2,500 GM, WELL	<2,500 GM, SICK
Bilirubin, mg/dl	20–24	15–20	10–15
Albumin	Alb (gm/dl) × 6.5	Alb (gm/dl) × 6.0	Alb (gm/dl) × 4.5
AUBC*	>20 nmol/L	>20 nmol/L	>15 nmol/L
Clinical	Symptomatic	Symptomatic	Deterioration
ABR	Abnormal	Deterioration	Deterioration†
Hematofluorometer‡	...	...	...

*"Alarm" level is *total* bilirubin concentration at which unbound bilirubin concentration (AUBC) reaches 20 nmol/L (if arterial pH >7.3). Binding is more likely to fluctuate in sick infants, and binding tests should be repeated daily in these infants.

†Baseline auditory brain-stem response (ABR) may be abnormal in sick or very premature infants.

‡"Alarm" level: total bilirubin level greater than total albumin-binding capacity (not validated by controlled study).

TABLE 30–3.—ACCEPTABLE INDICATIONS FOR PHOTOTHERAPY

BASIS	>2,500 GM	<2,500 GM, WELL	<2,500 GM, SICK
Bilirubin, mg/dl	15	10	7–8
Binding peroxidase	60% "alarm" level	50% "alarm" level	40–50% "alarm" level
Fluorometer	40% of total albumin-binding capacity (all groups)		

concentration [AUBC], automated peroxidase method) in our nursery.

b. There is reasonable intertest agreement between the peroxidase method, Sephadex filtration, and front-face fluorometry, although considerable disagreement is sometimes observed at high serum bilirubin levels.

c. Binding tests do not preclude the need for clinical judgment in managing the jaundiced infant.

4. Bilirubin may produce alterations in the auditory brain-stem response (ABR), including heightened threshold and prolonged I-III and I-V wave intervals, before clinical manifestations of toxic reaction become apparent.

5. Clinical signs of early kernicterus remain an absolute indication for exchange transfusion in any jaundiced infant.

6. Generally accepted indirect (unconjugated) serum bilirubin levels for exchange transfusion are shown in Table 30–2. (These guidelines were established primarily by consensus rather than by controlled studies, but have medical and legal precedent.)

E. PREVENTION OF HYPERBILIRUBINEMIA

1. Phototherapy

a. Indications for phototherapy have not been well established (Table 30–3). It is *not* an alternative to exchange transfusion when evidence of kernicterus or elevated unbound bilirubin is present.

2. Phenobarbital Is Not Recommended Except In Severe Hemolytic Disease.

31

Hemolytic Disease of the Newborn (HDN, Erythroblastosis Fetalis)

Erythroblastosis fetalis is usually due to sensitization of an Rh-negative woman by the red cells of an Rh-positive fetus, but severe hemolytic disease may be caused by maternal sensitization to many red cell antigens including little c, A, and Kell. Anemia, hyperbilirubinemia, or both may result in fetal or neonatal demise.

A. PREVENTION

Rh immune globulin (300 mg) is indicated only in nonsensitized Rh(D) negative women and given as follows:

1. Within 72 hours of delivery (about 98% effective), and at 28 weeks' gestation (combined therapy 99% effective).

2. After therapeutic abortion, amniocentesis, and abdominal trauma.

   In the latter case, Kleihauer-Betke acid elution test for fetal cells in maternal circulation should be obtained and volume of transfusion estimated. The RH immune globulin dose is 300 mg per 30 ml of fetal blood.

B. PRENATAL MANAGEMENT OF A SENSITIZED WOMAN

1. The timing of the delivery is based on history of previous pregnancy outcomes, antibody titers, serial amniocentesis, and ultrasound.

2. Measure anti-D antibodies on the first prenatal visit and peri-

odically through pregnancy (four-week intervals during the third trimester).

a. If the titer is greater than 1:32 (1:16 if previously immunized) perform amniocentesis at 26 to 28 weeks' gestation to evaluate the concentration of bilirubinoid pigments in the amniotic fluid (change in optical density at 450 nm [ΔOD_{450}], Figure 31–1).

b. If the antibody titer is higher, perform initial amniocentesis at 22 to 24 weeks' gestation.

3. Amniocentesis

a. The change in optical density at 450 nm provides a reasonably good prediction of anemia or risk of fetal death, but is less accurate in predicting the postnatal course of hyperbilirubinemia (Fig 31–1).

b. If the initial amniocentesis indicates that the fetus is moderately affected, the procedure should be repeated at two- to three-week intervals in order to monitor ΔOD_{450} and the L/S ratio.

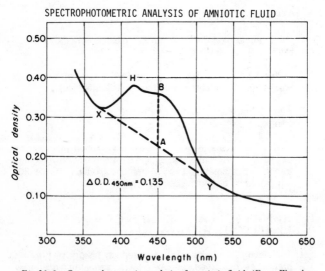

SPECTROPHOTOMETRIC ANALYSIS OF AMNIOTIC FLUID

Δ O.D. 450nm = 0.135

Fig 31–1.—Spectrophotometric analysis of amniotic fluid. (From Wennberg R.P., Krivit W.: Isoimmune hemolytic disease of the newborn, in Kelley V. (ed.): Brenneman-Kelley Textbook of Pediatrics. Hagerstown, Maryland, Harper & Row, 1972. Used by permission.)

c. If the ΔOD_{450} plots in zone III (Fig 31–2) or fails to decrease with advancing gestational age, we generally recommend the following:

  i. If the fetus is less than 30 weeks' gestation, perform intra-uterine transfusion with O Rh negative frozen deglycerized RBCs.

  ii. If the fetus has evidence of hydrops by ultrasound or amniography and is over 28 to 29 weeks' gestation, administer betamethasone (12 mg/day times two) to the mother (if the lung profile is immature) and deliver the infant.

  iii. If the fetus is severely affected (high zone II or zone III) and the lung profile is mature, administer phenobarbital

INTERPRETATION OF AMNIOTIC FLUID ANALYSIS

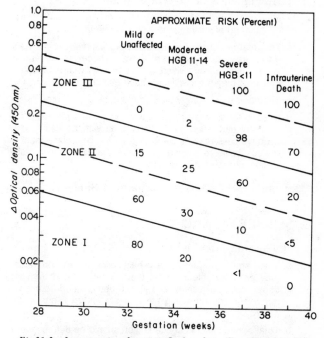

Fig 31–2.—*Interpretation of amniotic fluid analysis. (From Wennberg R.P., Krivit W.: Isoimmune hemolytic disease of the newborn, in Kelley V. (ed.): Brenneman-Kelley Textbook of Pediatrics. Hagerstown, Maryland, Harper & Row, 1972. Used by permission.)*

(125 mg/day) to the mother for three to seven days before delivery to stimulate the fetal hepatic conjugating system.

4. If amniocentesis indicates that the fetus is severely affected, tightly packed type O cells compatible with the mother's blood should be available at the time of delivery. These may be later mixed with AB plasma to reconstitute as whole blood if immediate red cell exchange is not needed for neonatal distress.

C. DELIVERY ROOM MANAGEMENT

1. Establish Ventilation and Stabilize Temperature.

2. Resuscitation of a Hydropic Infant

a. Minimize oxygen consumption by drying the infant and maintain an effective thermal environment.

b. The infant may require assisted ventilation with high inspiratory pressures. Paracentesis may be necessary to remove excess ascitic fluid, which, in combination with heptosplenomegaly, may mechanically impair effective ventilation.

c. Thoracentesis is rarely needed in the delivery room.

d. In severely hydropic or pale and asphyxiated infants, a 20- to 40-ml partial exchange transfusion with packed type O negative cells may be performed as the final component of the resuscitative procedure. Immediate exchange transfusion is otherwise not advised.

3. Obtain Cord Blood for Laboratory Studies.

D. NURSERY CARE

1. Laboratory Monitoring

a. The hematocrit (and occasionally bilirubin) in cord blood may be quite different from the values obtained from the baby after stabilization, and should be repeated from a venapuncture or indwelling catheter at 1 hour of age in the nursery.

b. Total serum bilirubin concentration should be determined at four- to six-hour intervals until the concentration declines.

c. Monitor direct bilirubin periodically for development of "inspissated bile syndrome."

2. **Phototherapy** has little effect on the early bilirubin rise, but may be useful in decreasing the number of exchange transfusions required.

3. **Indications for Early Exchange Transfusion** are found in Table 31–1.

4. **Indications for Later Exchange Transfusion** are similar to nonhemolytic jaundice.

5. **Other Problems**

   a. Hyaline membrane disease.

   b. In hydropic infants, severe cardiac arrhythmias may occur.

   c. Hypoglycemia (secondary to hyperinsulinemia).

   d. Erythroblastotic infants may have low folate levels; consider folate supplementation.

TABLE 31–1.—CRITERIA FOR EXCHANGE TRANSFUSION IN ERYTHROBLASTOSIS FETALIS*

All patients
　Cord hemoglobin <8 gm/dl
　Cord bilirubin concentration >6 mg/dl
　Two hour bilirubin concentration >7.5 mg/dl
　Rise in bilirubin at 2–12 hr of age >0.5 mg/dl/hr
Uncomplicated HDN
　Indirect bilirubin concentration >20 mg/dl
　Indirect bilirubin concentration (in mg/dl) >6.5 × albumin
　　concentration (gm/dl)
　AUBC (peroxidase method) 15–20 nmol/L (if arterial pH 7.3–
　　7.5)
　Sephadex staining 1+ (kernlute)
Complicated HDN (e.g., HMD, hydrops)
　Indirect bilirubin concentration (in mg/dl) 4.4–5.5 × albumin
　　concentration (in gm/dl) (lower range for sick babies who had
　　prenatal asphyxia or who are vulnerable to acidosis, e.g.,
　　HMD)
　AUBC (peroxidase) 10–15 nmol (if pH 7.1–7.3)
　Sephadex staining 1+ (Kernlute)
Clinical deterioration
　Irritability, lethargy, development of abnormal brain-stem
　　auditory evoked response

*HDN indicates hemolytic disease of the newborn; HMD, hyaline membrane disease; AUBC, apparent unbound bilirubin concentration.

e. Thrombocytopenia.

f. Obstructive jaundice may result from bilirubin overload to the liver (conjugated bilirubin appears) or liver bilirubin toxicity (inspissated bile syndrome).

g. Delayed anemia (at 3 to 4 months of age) is common, especially when exchange transfusion is not required.

32

Conjugated Hyperbilirubinemia in Neonates

A. DEFINITION

A direct bilirubin concentration greater than 1.5 mg/dl is the minimal diagnostic criterion. It is *always* pathological.

B. MECHANISMS

1. **Hepatocellular Injury** due to infections, shock, toxins, metabolic disorders, drugs, and "neonatal hepatitis."

2. **Obstruction of Bile Flow** due to extrahepatic and intrahepatic biliary atresia, choledochal cyst, "inspissated bile," and other cholestatis syndromes.

3. **Increased Bilirubin Loading** due to acute hemolytic disease, multiple blood transfusions.

4. **Congenital Disorders of Bilirubin Excretion** (Dubin-Johnson syndrome, Rotor's syndrome).

C. DIAGNOSTIC CONSIDERATIONS

1. Clinical

a. "Sick" infant. Sudden development of direct bilirubinemia may be due to hepatocellular injury from the following:
   i. Shock
   ii. Sepsis (bacterial, viral, fungal)
   iii. Metabolic disorders

b. "Sick" infant with onset of symptoms after feeding suggests metabolic disease:
   i. Galactosemia (if fed breast milk or cow's milk formula)

ii. Fructosemia (if fed Nutramigen or soy formula with sucrose, e.g., Isomil)

c. Nonacute illness in an infant with prolonged jaundice and elevated direct bilirubin level may be caused by the following:
   i. Neonatal hepatitis
   ii. Extrahepatic biliary atresia
   iii. Choledochal cyst
   iv. Intrahepatic paucity of bile ducts (Biliary hypoplasia)
   v. α-1-antitrypsin deficiency
   vi. Cystic fibrosis
   vii. Hypothyroidism
   viii. Cholestatis syndrome (inspissated bile, etc.)
   ix. Congenital defects of excretion

d. Infant receiving TPN (10% to 15%). This usually resolves with discontinuation of TPN, but cirrhosis has been reported.

D. DIAGNOSTIC EVALUATION

1. Routine Studies

a. Bilirubin concentration (total/direct) establishes the diagnosis of conjugated hyperbilirubinemia if the direct fraction is greater than 1.5 mg/dl. Measure the bilirubin concentration in the urine if there is a borderline elevation of direct fraction.

b. Transaminase (SGOT/SGPT) levels elevated two to three times normal suggests hepatocellular injury.

c. Alkaline phosphatase (ALK-PHOS) and gamma glutamyl transferase (GGT) values greater than two to three times normal may indicate intrahepatic or extrahepatic biliary obstruction.

d. Blood and urine cultures, TORCH titers, urine CMV cultures, skin scrapings for viral inclusions, HBsAG, and IgM-hepatitis A antibody determinations may indicate an infectious cause.

e. Serum α-1-antitrypsin levels lower than 100 mg/dl are diagnostic of α-1-antitrypsin deficiency. Confirm by phenotyping (PiZZ) and liver biopsy.

f. Complete blood cell count, reticulocyte counts, ABO, Coombs' test, and Rh determinations may suggest hemolytic disease with increased bilirubin loading or inspissated bile syndrome.

g. Urine Clinitest for reducing substances may be positive in galactosemia fructose intolerance and tyrosinosis.

h. Urine metabolic screen, if positve, may suggest tryosinosis or other aminoacidurias.

2. **"Second Level" Studies** are used to further define anatomic or metabolic abnormalities suggested by routine studies:

   a. Neonatal T_4, TSH, and uridine diphosphogalactose studies confirm or help to eliminate hypothyroidism or galactosemia.

   b. Serum and urine amino acids for tyrosinosis or other aminoacidurias.

   c. Quantitative sweat chloride for cystic fibrosis.

   d. Fructose tolerance test for fructose intolerance.

   e. Ultrasound of liver and biliary tract may define normal or absent extrahepatic ducts, gallbladder, or presence of a choledochal cyst.

   f. Biliary scan following three to five days of phenobarbital loading (5 mg/kg/day) may demonstrate patency of biliary system. (CAUTION: Severe cholestasis may prevent excretion of the isotope into the GI tract; experience to date suggests this study is helpful only if the result is positive.)

   g. Quantitative rose bengal sodium I 131 excretion study with stool collections suggests biliary atresia if less than 5% to 10% of the administered dose is excreted over 72 hours.

3. **"Third Level" Studies** are done for unexplained hyperbilirubinemia or for evaluation of possible biliary atresia.

   a. Percutaneous liver biopsy may define hepatocellular disease (e.g., neonatal hepatitis) or suggest anatomic obstruction (biliary hypoplasia, biliary atresia).

   b. Percutaneous cholangiogram, if successful, may define normal or abnormal biliary tract anatomy.

   c. Operative cholangiogram is indicated where the diagnosis of biliary atresia or choledochal cyst is suspected.

E. THERAPY

Therapy for the infant with liver disease and conjugated hyperbilirubinemia is directed at supportive care, removing offending toxins, relieving anatomic obstructions, increasing bile flow, and providing adequate nutrition.

33

Hypoglycemia

A. INFANTS AT RISK

1. **Infants of Diabetic Mothers** Onset may occur as early as 1 to 2 hours of age.

2. **Fetal Malnutrition, SGA**

3. **Severe Asphyxia**

4. **Rh hemolytic disease (hyperinsulinism)**

5. **Polycythemia**

6. **Fasted Stressed Infants**

7. **Syndromes**
   a. Beckwith's syndrome (probable hyperinsulinism)
   b. Microphallus (Look for other signs of hypopituitarism.)

8. **Inherited Metabolic Disease**
   a. Galactosemia, Fructose Intolerance
   b. Pyruvate Carboxylase Deficiency
   c. Glycogen Storage Disease

9. **Tumors**
   a. Insulinoma
   b. Nesidioblastosis

10. Infiltration or cessation of high rate or glucose infusion (e.g., TPN) without immediately restarting IV

B. SYMPTOMS

1. May begin within a few hours of age or as late as 1 week of age.

2. There is often a time lag between onset of hypoglycemia and symptoms.

3. Seizures are associated with a high incidence of poor neurological outcome.

4. Other symptoms associated with hypoglycemia include lethargy, poor feeding, apathy, changes in tone, cyanosis (pulmonary hypertension), and apnea. These symptoms have been reported with low blood glucose values and respond to administration of glucose.

C. DIAGNOSIS

1. **Asymptomatic Hypoglycemia**

   a. Suspect when Dextrostix result is less than 45 mg/dl.

   b. Order STAT quantitative blood sugar.

   c. Diagnosis is indicated when the blood sugar level is less than 30 mg/dl in a term infant, and less than 20 mg/dl in a preterm infant.

2. **Symptomatic Hypoglycemia** is defined as symptoms that disappear with glucose infusion regardless of blood glucose.

D. SAMPLE COLLECTION AND ANALYSIS

1. Screen with Dextrostix within 15 minutes of birth if an infant of a diabetic mother or if suspicious of hypoglycemia. Repeat every 15 to 30 minutes until dextrostix remains constant.

2. Samples must be collected in fluoride tubes to prevent unpredictable glucose utilization by erythrocytes.

E. THERAPY

1. Always Draw Quantitative Blood Glucose Prior to Treatment

2. Asymptomatic Infant

a. Start oral feedings with 10% dextrose in water or formula orally or by gavage.

b. If oral intake is unsuccessful, start IV to deliver 5 to 7 mg/kg/min of glucose.

3. Symptomatic or Suspected Symptomatic Infant

a. Start an IV push of 1 ml/kg of 25% glucose (250 mg/kg).

b. Start continuous infusion, 7 to 10 mg/kg/min of glucose.

4. Increase glucose infusion rate as necessary to maintain a Dextrostix reading greater than 45 mg/dl.

5. Monitor glucose level every 15 minutes until it is stable and adjust IV to maintain blood glucose level in the 60- to 90-mg/dl range. Some infants may require up to 10 to 20 mg/kg/min. Avoid hyperglycemia.

6. To decide the initial IV rate given a desired glucose infusion rate (r, mg/kg/min), use equation A. If the glucose infusion is to be calculated at given IV rates, use equation B.
   A. IV rate in ml/hr = $6 \times r \times$ wt in kg/% glucose in IV solution
   B. r = (IV rate in ml/hr)(% glucose in IV solution)/($6 \times$ wt in kg)

7. Taper IV rate while monitoring blood glucose level. If IV comes out, IT MUST BE RESTARTED IMMEDIATELY, especially in infants who have been receiving prolonged high glucose infusions.

8. Monitor glucose level every four to six hours for one day after hypoglycemia is resolved.

9. Other Therapies

a. Glucagon, 300 μg/kg up to 1 mg. Effective in IDMs. Not effective in SGA babies with low glycogen stores and impaired gluconeogenesis.

b. Steroids are used in intractable hypoglycemia, usually in SGA infants, and only under the guidance of the attending physician.

c. Surgery is rarely indicated.

d. Susphrine or epinephrine may produce lactic acidosis and are not recommended.

F. PROGNOSIS

1. Transient asymptomatic hypoglycemia as seen with asphyxia or IDMs is associated with good outcome.

2. Symptomatic hypoglycemia is associated with poor neurological outcome.

3. SGA infants have a high incidence of hypoglycemia as well as poor neurological outcome.

34

Endocrine Problems

A. CONGENITAL HYPOTHYROIDISM

Physical stigmata of congenital hypothyroidism in the newborn are too subtle for physical diagnosis in most cases. The prevalence and morbidity, including mental retardation, if not treated, are sufficient to make screening cost effective. Thus, most states currently require newborn screening for hypothyroidism. The sooner the treatment is started, the better the ultimate intelligence in the child.

1. **Incidence** One in 4,000 live births.

2. **Screening** Measurement of T_4 concentration is done on spot of blood. Those concentrations below the 95% confidence levels of the laboratory will also have a TSH measurement done.

3. **Diagnosis (Fig. 34–1)**

   a. Primary hypothyroidism is indicated by a low T_4 and elevated TSH level.

   b. A low T_4 level may be accompanied by a normal TSH value, which may indicate a physiologically normal thyroid status but a low concentration of thyroid-binding globulin (TBG). This is frequently seen in premature infants and confirmed by finding a normal free thyroxin level. Alternatively, a low T_4 with a normal TSH value may indicate hypopituitarism or hypothalamic deficiency, and further diagnostic measures may be required.

   c. An iodinated I^{123} or technetium scan of the thyroid is indicated to evaluate the presence of a rudimentary or ectopic thyroid only if the scanning facility has adequate experience with newborns. Scans must be performed prior to therapy.

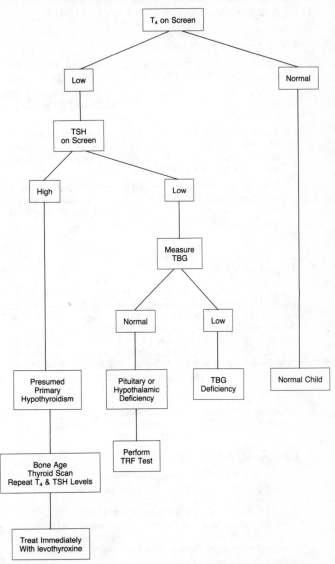

Fig 34–1.—Algorithm for diagnosis of primary hypothyroidism. T₄ indicates serum thyroxine; TSH, thyroid-stimulating hormone; TBG, thyroid-binding globulin; TRF, thyrotropin-releasing factor.

4. Treatment   Levothyroxine

a. Levothyroxine is administered at 5 to 10 μg/kg. Tablets are crushed and administered orally.

b. Do not withhold treatment for the confirmation results; as long as the samples for the repeated T_4 and TSH studies have been sent, therapy should begin.

c. Serum T_4 is measured after five days of therapy and the thyroxine dosage adjusted on the basis of the T_4 concentration. The goal is to keep the serum T_4 value in the upper half of the normal range for age.

d. The TSH concentration may remain elevated for months in many patients because of immaturity of the feedback mechanism. Thus, adequate therapy cannot be assessed by monitoring TSH values.

B. AMBIGUOUS GENITALIA—INTERSEX PROBLEMS

Intersex problems must be considered psychosocial emergencies, and under no circumstances should the family be told the sex of the child until the diagnosis has been made. Only an experienced physician, usually a pediatric endocrinologist or neonatologist, should address this difficult problem. If only an encyclopedic discussion of the problem is carried out with the parents without regard for their invariably distressed emotional state, long-standing psychopathologic problems can result.

1. The patient could be a male pseudohermaphrodite (an XY individual with inadequate virilization), a female pseudohermaphrodite (an XX individual with excess virilization), or a true hermaphrodite (Table 34–1).

2. Diagnosis (Fig. 34–2)

a. Examine the patient for palpable gonads.
   i. If palpable, the patient has a greater chance of being a male pseudohermaphrodite.
   ii. If not palpable, the diagnosis is uncertain.
   iii. Rectal examination followed by ultrasound examination for cervix and uterus is useful. If the uterus is present, the patient is most likely a female pseudohermaphrodite.

b. Perform the following laboratory tests:
   i. Karyotype and, if laboratory has experience in the technique, a buccal smear for Barr bodies. (Buccal smear can

TABLE 34–1.—HERMAPHRODITISM

I. Female pseudohermaphroditism
   A. Congenital adrenal hyperplasia
      21 Hydroxylase deficiency (the most common cause)
      3 β-hydroxysteroid dehydrogenase deficiency
      11 Hydroxylase deficiency
   B. Maternal androgen administration
II. Male pseudohermaphroditism
   A. Enzymatic defects affecting the adrenal gland and the
      testes
      1. 20–22 desmolase deficiency
      2. 3 β-ol deficiency
      3. 17 α-hydroxylase deficiency
   B. Enzymatic defects affecting the testes
      1. 17,20 desmolase deficiency
      2. 17 β-oxidoreductase deficiency
   C. End-organ resistance to testosterone
      1. Syndrome of testicular feminization (complete)
      2. Syndrome of testicular ferminization (incomplete)
   D. Localized enzymatic defect in sexual skin
      5 α-reductase deficiency
   E. Dysgenetic testes
      1. Syndrome of gonadal dysgenesis (XO/XY)
      2. With XY karyotype
   F. Variants of the Klinefelter syndrome of seminiferous tubular
      dysgenesis (XXY, XXXY, etc.)
III. True hermaphroditism

---

be read within a few hours, but misinterpretation is possible.)

ii. Serum sodium and potassium levels will determine if salt
loss and potassium retention are occurring. (This usually
does not develop until the fifth to the seventh day of life.)

iii. Quantitative urinary collection for sodium and potassium
to assess salt loss.

iv. Plasma 17-hydroxy progesterone, dihydropiandrosterone,
dihydrotestosterone, testosterone, and androstenedione
and 11-hydroxy cortisol to determine if an enzymatic
block is present.

v. Urinary 17 KS, 17 OHCS, and pregnanetriol excretion will
often return sooner than the plasma samples listed in iv.

vi. Again, no matter what pressure is applied, no gender as-
signment can be made with inadequate evaluation. The
child should be referred to in neutral terms until that time.

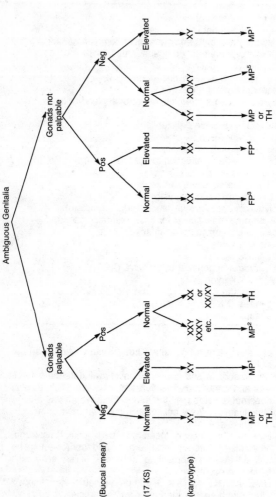

Fig 34–2.—Algorithm for diagnosis in cases of ambiguous genitalia. MP indicates male pseudohermaphroditism; FP, female pseudohermaphroditism; TH, true hermaphroditism.

Superscripts indicate the following: [1], congenital adrenal hyperplasia—3βol deficiency; [2], variants of seminiferous tubular dysgenesis; [3], not due to an adrenal defect; [4], due to an adrenal enzyme defect; [5], due to syndrome of gonadal dysgenesis with dysgenetic testes.

3. Treatment (Adrenal Insufficiency)

a. In the absence of endogenous cortisol, hypoglycemia and shock may result.
   i. The normal secretion rate of cortisol is 12.5 to 15 mg/sq mm/day, and therapy is directed to replace this amount.
   ii. Parenteral hydrocortisone (IV) at 12.5 mg/sq mm/day or cortisone acetate (IM) at 15 mg/sq mm/day are appropriate beginning doses.
   iii. Intravenous preparations are immediately effective, but quickly disappear and must be given every four to six hours in divided doses. Intramuscular cortisone acetate is not effective for several hours after adminstration and, therefore, cannot be used in an emergency.
   iv. Because it lasts three days, the most convenient regimen is triple the daily dose given every three days.

b. Mineralocorticoid therapy
   i. If salt loss has been documented, desoxycorticosterone acetate (DOCA) is given at about 1 mg/day IM.
   ii. Treatment with DOCA will not be effective unless sodium is administered. One gram of extra salt can be given orally, or normal saline may be used as the "maintenance" intravenous fluid if IV is being administered.
   iii. Salt retention and hypertension are a result of excessive dosage and excessive salt administration. Blood pressure should be monitored.

REFERENCE

1. Grumbach M.M., Conte F.A.: Disorders of sexual differentiation, in Williams R.H.: *Textbook of Endocrinology*. Philadelphia, W.B. Saunders Co., 1981.

35

Serious Inherited
Metabolic Disease

A. SUSPECT

1. Family history of early unexplained neonatal deaths.

2. Unexplained deterioration in clinical status.

3. Differential diagnosis of septic shock, coma, delayed renal failure, seizures, bleeding and hemolytic disorders, jaundice, unexplained metabolic acidosis.

B. DIAGNOSTIC SCREENING

1. **Serum** Sodium, potassium, bicarbonate, chloride, anion gap.

2. **Blood** pH, ammonia, lactate, ketones, glucose, BUN.

3. **Plasma (Heparinized)** Analyze 2 ml for amino and organic acid determination.

4. Urine metabolic screen, amino and organic acid analysis, microscopic examination for crystals.

C. TREATMENT—BASIC PRINCIPLES

1. **Maintain Maximum Calories to Prevent Catabolism.**

2. **Add Glucose, Fat, and Protein Sequentially.**

3. If the Patient Is Severely Ill

a. Attempt to remove toxic metabolites by exchange transfusion, hemodialysis, or peritoneal dialysis.

b. Provide high concentrations of B vitamins.

D. IF THE PATIENT IS DYING

1. Premortem Save 3 to 5 ml of heparinized blood, 3 to 5 ml of unheparinized blood, and 5 to 10 ml of urine.

a. Separate RBCs (for enzyme studies) and plasma (for toxins).

b. Refrigerate RBCs.

c. Freeze urine, plasma, and serum specimen at $-20°C$ ($-70°C$ preferred).

2. Postmortem examination must be performed immediately after death. The need for immediate examination usually must be discussed with the parents before death occurs.

a. Obtain a skin biopsy for fibroblast culture.
   i. Prepare skin and use sterile technique.
   ii. Place in viral culture media (nutrients plus antibiotics).

b. Obtain tissue samples, 1 to 5 gm of liver, muscle, kidney, brain.
   i. For enzyme analysis, freeze immediately in liquid nitrogen or in isopentane chilled on dry ice and stored at $-70°C$.
   ii. For electron microscopy (EM) studies, fix fresh tissue in glutaraldehyde.

E. SPECIFIC DISORDERS SEEN IN THE NEWBORN PERIOD

1. Transient Hyperammonemia (Cause Unknown)

a. *Usual presentation* Most cases are larger premature infants weighing 1,500 to 2,500 gm who have respiratory distress. Lethargy progresses to coma, decorticate or decerebrate posturing, and seizures. Oliguria and sclerema are common. Hyperammonemia may reach over 3,000 mg/dl, usually peaking by the third to fifth day of life.

b. *Diagnosis* Suspect this disorder in a newborn with a rapidly rising ammonia level in the absence of protein load. Diagnosis is confirmed by rapid resolution.

c. *Treatment* Ventilatory support is usually required. The rise in ammonia may be modified by repeated exchange transfusions, peritoneal dialysis, or hemodialysis. Maintain low protein intake. Administer sodium benzoate, 200 mg IV followed by a continuous infusion of 200 to 400 mg/kg/day if the serum bilirubin concentration is low (controversial). The disease usually resolves spontaneously by 2 weeks of age.

d. *Outcome* Short-term follow-up of survivors suggests normal growth and development.

2. Hyperammonemia Due to Urea Cycle Enzyme Deficiencies

a. *Usual presentation* Periodic vomiting, lethargy, and CNS signs leading to coma, seizures, or both. May mimic transient hyperammonemia, but onset is usually more gradual and related to the quantity of protein intake. When symptoms present in the newborn, the defect is usually lethal.

b. *Diagnosis* Suspect this disorder if the blood ammonia level is greater than 300 mg/dl and rises progressively with continued feeding. Obtain plasma and urine amino acid levels to identify elevations in Krebs cycles intermediates and urine orotic acid.

c. *Etiology* Four urea cycle enzymes have been reported to produce overwhelming disease in the newborn:
   i. Ornithine transcarbamylase: sex linked and lethal in males.
   ii. Carbamyl phosphate synthetase: citrullinemia (argininosuccinic acid synthetase), and argininosuccinic aciduria (friable hair) are probably autosomal recessive.

d. *Treatment* Emergency treatment as in transient hyperammonemia. Maintain low protein intake. Administer a special diet containing low protein and α-keto analogues of amino acids.

3. Lactic Acidosis With Hypoglycemia

a. *Usual presentation* Symptoms are related to hypoglycemia and tachypnea.

b. *Diagnosis* Hypoglycemia and lactic acidosis are responsive to glucose infusion. If the infant is receiving formula containing sucrose suspect fructose intolerance. If he is taking a milk formula suspect galactosemia (rarely a cause of severe hypoglycemia). Perform a liver biopsy for morphological findings and enzyme assay. Do a glucagon tolerance test.

c. *Etiology* Elevated lactate level is secondary to block in gluconeogenesis. The most common causes are as follows:

  i. Glycogen storage disease type I (Gaucher's disease): glucose-6-phosphatase deficiency.

  ii. Fructose intolerance: aldolase B deficiency.

  iii. Fructose-1,6-diphosphatase deficiency.

  iv. Phospho-enol pyruvate kinase deficiency.

d. *Treatment* Fructose-free diet in aldolase B deficiency. Glucose-based diet in type I storage disease.

e. *Outcome* Variable; requires early and aggressive treatment.

4. Lactic Acidosis Without Hypoglycemia

a. *Usual presentation* In severe forms, patients are SGA, often with minor congenital defects, microcephalic with large ventricles, compensated severe metabolic acidosis (often alkalotic if corrected with bicarbonate), frequently premature, and they fail to grow. Milder forms may simply have lethargy and are frequently asymptomatic unless stressed with a high carbohydrate load or illness.

b. *Diagnosis* Lactic acidosis worsens on high carbohydrate load, and improves on a high-fat low-carbohydrate diet. Specific enzyme assay on skin or liver biopsy.

c. *Etiology* Most often involves primary or secondary blocks in either pyruvate carboxylase or the pyruvate dehydrogenase complex.

d. *Treatment* If secondary, treat the underlying defect. If primary, a high-fat low-carbohydrate diet may ameliorate lactic acidosis and symptoms, but will not significantly alter prognosis in infants affected prenatally. Megavitamin treatment with thiamine and biotin may be helpful.

e. *Outcome* Microcephaly, failure to thrive, or severe mental retardation is inevitable in severe deficiencies.

5. Maple Syrup Urine Disease Branched chain aminoaciduria involving leucine, isoleucine, valine.

a. *Usual presentation* Apathy, hypertonia or hypotonia, and tonic seizures often in association with hypoglycemia. Death occurs without treatment. The typical maple syrup odor may not be present.

b. *Diagnosis* Alpha-keto organic acids in urine are detected by 2,4-dinitrophenylhydrazine. Branched-chain amino acid levels are elevated in plasma.

c. *Etiology* Defect in metabolism of branched chains and their keto acid analogues. Autosomal recessive.

d. *Treatment* High-dose thiamine trial (most forms not responsive). Dietary restriction. Peritoneal dialysis.

e. *Outcome* Guarded prognosis for life or normal development.

6. **Disorders of Propionic Acid Metabolism** Propionic acidemia, ketotic hyperglycinemia, methylmalonic acidemia.

a. *Usual presentation* Lethargy, vomiting, profound metabolic acidosis, coma. In less severe forms, failure to thrive, vomiting, and mild acidosis are seen.

b. *Diagnosis* Large anion gap, ketoacidosis, hyperammonemia (occasionally), hyperglycinemia, elevated branched-chain amino acid levels. Elevated methylmalonic acid or propionic acid levels differentiate the three conditions. Enzyme deficiency detected in WBCs or liver.

c. *Treatment* Restrict protein. One form of methylmalonic acidemia responds to high doses of cofactor vitamin B_{12}.

d. *Outcome* Most patients do poorly and have mental retardation. Death usually occurs in the newborn period or with exacerbations.

7. **Nonketotic Hyperglycinemia**

a. *Usual presentation* Profound neurological signs characterized by hypotonia, lethargy, poor feeding, coma, seizures, apnea. About one third of the patients die in the first two weeks.

b. *Diagnosis* Plasma glycine level is increased two to 20 times normal.

c. *Etiology* Block in the glycine cleavage system to form methyl tetrahydrofolic acid. Mechanism of profound CNS signs is unknown.

d. *Treatment* No effective therapy is known, although methionine and sodium benzoate may reduce the plasma glycine level.

e. *Outcome* About one third of the patients die in the first two weeks. Severe brain damage and early death usually result.

REFERENCES

1. Danks D.M.: Management of newborn babies in whom serious metabolic illness is anticipated. *Arch. Dis. Child.* 49:556, 1974.
2. Nyhan W.L.: An approach to the diagnosis of overwhelming metabolic disease in early infancy. *Current Problems in Pediatrics* 7:3–20, 1977.

36

Congenital Anomalies and Genetic Disorders

A. DEFINITIONS AND CLASSIFICATIONS

1. **Congenital Anomalies** Abnormalities of shape, structure, or both are present before parturition.

   a. Classification by cause
      i. Acquired (e.g., thalidomide).
      ii. Genetic (e.g., Down's syndrome, albinism).
      iii. Combination (e.g., polygenic/multifactorial).
      iv. Unknown (e.g., amniotic band disruption).

   b. Classification by pathogenesis
      i. Malformation: primary structural defect.
      ii. Deformation: secondary alterations.
      iii. Disruption.

   c. Classification by grouping pattern
      i. Syndromes: multiple malformations in one or more tissues in recurrent combinations and believed due to a single cause (e.g., Down's syndrome, rubella syndrome).
      ii. Sequences: combination of primary malformation and secondary deformation (e.g., Robin's sequence).
      iii. Associations: nonrandom clusters of malformations not clearly syndromes or sequences (e.g., Vater syndrome).

2. **Genetic Disorders** Abnormalities due to changes in the genes or chromosomes.

   a. Single major gene (dominant, recessive, x-linked).

   b. Polygenic—multifactorial.

   c. Chromosomal (trisomies, deletions, translocations, inversions, mosaics).
      i. Prior to conception (nonmosaic).
      ii. After conception (chromosome mosaics).

B. MAJOR ANOMALIES

1. **Incidence**   Five percent (one in 20) births have significant (major) anomalies, genetic disorders, or both. Some are undetectable until later.

2. **Evaluation**

   a. Physical/functional description. Subtle anomalies may be clues to the diagnosis of a specific syndrome or to the presence of a hidden nonspecific major abnormality.

   b. Assess the cause through history of fetal environment and family pedigree (successful in about one half the cases).
      i. Pregnancy history for toxins, disease, irradiation.
      ii. Eliminate in utero insult and if any anomaly had its embryologic origin prior to the time of the alleged insult.
      iii. The family pedigree should be obtained using a standard technique.

C. MINOR ANOMALIES

   These include true abnormalities that are mild enough not to be considered of medical or cosmetic consequence.

1. **Incidence**

   a. Minor anomalies in less than 10% of the general population.

   b. Minor anomalies may be an important clue to the presence of a hidden, associated major anomaly.

2. **Evaluation**

   a. A minor anomaly loses its potential significance when it is observed to be a familial trait in other normal relatives.

   b. Measurable gradations from too little to too much should be plotted against standardized norms, e.g., head size, distance between nipples, etc. (Table 36–1).

D. CHROMOSOMAL ANOMALIES

1. **Incidence**   One in approximately 150 live-born babies has a detectable chromosomal abnormality.

   a. Less than 10% of babies with congenital anomalies have detectable chromosome abnormalities, and most of these involve the autosomes.

TABLE 36–1.—Listing of Normal Full-Term Newborn Measurements*

	MEAN	+2nd STANDARD DEVIATION (+2)	–2nd STANDARD DEVIATION (–2)
Body weight	7.5 lb (3.4 kg)	9.7 lb (4.3 kg)	5.8 lb (2.6 kg)
Body length	19.9 in (50.5 cm)	21.6 in (54.8 cm)	18.3 in (46.5 cm)
Head circumference	13.5 in (34.4 cm)	14.6 in (37.0 cm)	12.6 in (32.0 cm)
Anterior fontanelle diameter	0.8 in (0.2 cm)	1.6 in (4.0 cm)	0.4 in (1.0 cm)
Posterior fontanelle diameter	0.2 in (0.5 cm)	0.4 in (1.0 cm)	0.1 in (0.2 cm)
Chest circumference	12.8 in (32.5 cm)	14.7 in (37.4 cm)	11.0 in (28.0 cm)
Internipple distance	3.3 in (8.3 cm)	3.9 in (10.0 cm)	2.6 in (6.6 cm)
Hand length	2.6 in (6.6 cm)	3.1 in (7.8 cm)	2.2 in (5.5 cm)
Middle finger length	1.1 in (2.8 cm)	1.4 in (3.5 cm)	0.9 in (2.2 cm)
Palm length	1.5 in (3.8 cm)	1.9 in (4.7 cm)	1.1 in (2.9 cm)
Interpupil distance	1.5 in (3.9 cm)	1.8 in (4.5 cm)	1.3 in (3.3 cm)
Inner canthal distance	0.8 in (2.0 cm)	1.0 in (2.5 cm)	0.6 in (1.5 cm)
Outer canthal distance	2.5 in (6.3 cm)	2.9 in (7.3 cm)	2.1 in (5.3 cm)
Ear length	1.4 in (3.5 cm)	1.7 in (4.2 cm)	1.1 in (2.9 cm)
Penis length (stretched)	1.6 in (4.0 cm)	2.2 in (5.5 cm)	1.3 in (3.2 cm)
Upper (crown-symphysis) to lower (symphysis-heel) ratio	1.7/1	1.9/1	1.5/1

Low-set ears: When the upper anterior attachment of the helix is below a horizontal line extending from the medial canthus through the lateral canthus of the eye.

Rotated ears: When the angle of slope of the ear is greater than 10° from the perpendicular.

Small recessed chin: When apex of chin is posterior to a vertical line through the corner of the mouth.

Prominent forehead: When forehead protrudes anterior to a vertical line through the bridge of the medial eyebrow.

*From Smith D.W., Siegel J.D.: Recognizable patterns of human malformations, in Markowitz M. (ed.): *Major Problems in Clinical Pediatrics,* Vol. II. Philadelphia, W. B. Saunders Co., 1982. Used by permission.

b. Balanced translocations, and most inversions as well as most sex chromosome aberrations, e.g., variations of XXY, XXX, and XYY, may not present with congenital malformations.

2. Indications for Chromosome Analysis in Infants With Congenital Anomalies

a. Any obvious suspected chromosomal syndrome (Down's syndrome, Turner's syndrome, etc.) to verify the diagnosis and distinguish the different possible forms (trisomies, translocations, mosaics).

b. Multiple anomalies not identifiable as an established single gene syndrome.

c. Unusual-looking facies unlike other members of the family. These usually are a composite of multiple minor malformations, each of no consequence by itself.

d. Ambiguous genitalia.

E. GENETIC COUNSELING

1. Parents should be encouraged to view and interact with their infant.

2. Counseling and description of anomalies should be done in comprehensible lay terms and in a timely manner.

3. Risks of recurrence should be explained as soon as known.

4. Follow-up counseling to clarify initial explanation, answer questions, reiterate recurrence risks, and discuss implications for family planning should be accomplished by the primary physician and a medical geneticist or social worker.

REFERENCES

1. Bergsma D. (ed.): *Birth Defects Compendium,* National Foundation-March of Dimes, ed 2. New York, Alan R. Liss, 1979.
2. Smith D.W., Jones K.L.: *Genetic, Embryologic and Clinical Aspects Recognizable Patterns of Human Malformation,* ed. 3. Philadephia, W.B. Saunders Co., 1982, p. 45.

37

Death and Dying

A. BEFORE DEATH

1. The parents need:

   a. Information that their baby is in critical condition.

   b. Knowledge of factors contributing to a positive or negative outcome.

   c. Human contact with the baby (if desired) including feeding or simple nursing tasks.

   d. Participation in decision making re: procedures, life-support measures, holding their baby, baptism, when death is imminent, etc.

2. The attending and resident physicians need to:

   a. Address ethical issues re: continuance of life support. Realize that opinions are mixed and strongly held (i.e., preserve life at all costs vs. death with dignity). Receive consultation from hospital/nursery ethics committee when appropriate.

   b. Be committed to the process of talking with the parents and be their professional "guide." Let them discuss which way they want to go, give your professional opinion of pros and cons of each option, accompany and support them once a decision has been made.

   c. Coordinate the involvement of the health care team.

3. The health care team needs to:

   a. Identify personal feelings that "this child might die."

   b. Meet, negotiate roles, and identify team members who can provide primary support to the parents.

B. IMMEDIATELY AFTER DEATH

1. Be aware of stages of grieving: shock, inertia, disorganization, volatile emotions, guilt, loss and loneliness, relief, re-establishment (may not necessarily occur in sequence, and may take two to six months to resolve).

2. The physician needs to succinctly explain the cause of death (best with parents together, but don't delay if one is not available), and help prepare time and place for grieving to take place. Share the normality of grief stages, including physical reactions such as crying, poor concentration, sleeplessness and anxiety.

   a. Realize that parents' frustration or anger is part of the process.

   b. Encourage expression of feelings ("It may be useful to talk"), but don't force them ("You must be feeling----").

   c. Expect a variety of emotional responses.

   d. Establish the need for autopsy.

   e. Parents should be encouraged to share their grief with each other, with their families, and with their friends.

   f. Mothers should be encouraged to grieve in their own way, make their needs known if still a patient, and carefully consider all decisions concerning the baby.

   g. Fathers should be encouraged to grieve in their own way; men may need "permission" to express their feelings (male friends or physicians can help "open up" this process), and share them with their spouses.

C. ONE TO TWO MONTHS AFTER DEATH

1. A follow-up visit with the attending physician and/or the family physician (if possible) should:

   a. Present a concise summary of medical events leading to the child's death.

   b. Explore ongoing grieving. Are feelings being shared between parents, siblings, and other family members? Are there family or social barriers which prevent appropriate grieving?

    c. Review autopsy findings.

    d. Arrange genetic counseling if needed and not already scheduled.

REFERENCES

1. Kennell J.H., et al.: The mourning responses of parents to the death of a newborn infant. *N. Engl. J. Med.* 284:349, 1970.
2. Peppers L.G., Knapp R.J.: *Motherhood and Mourning—Perinatal Death.* New York, Praeger, 1980.
3. Schweibert P., Kirk P.: *When Hello Means Goodbye: A Guide for Parents Whose Child Dies at Birth or Shortly After.* Portland, OR, University of Oregon Health Sciences Center, 1981.
4. Solnit A.J., Green M.: Psychologic considerations in the management of deaths on pediatric hospital services. I. The doctor and the child's family. *Pediatrics* 24(1):106–112, 1959.

38

Oxygen Therapy

Supplemental oxygen is an important form of therapy for many infants with cardiopulmonary disorders. It should be recognized that its use may be associated with the occurrence of retrolental fibroplasia and chronic lung disease and that criteria have not been established that ensure minimal hazard to the patient. Therefore, we presently recommend that oxygen administration be regulated to maintain the arterial Po_2 within the range for normal newborns, 50 to 100 torr.

A. INDICATIONS

1. **Hypoxemia** Hypoxemia in the newborn is usually defined as a Pa_{O_2} less than 50 torr.

2. **Resuscitation** Some practitioners recommend limitation of FI_{O_2} to 0.80 for resuscitation in the delivery room.

3. **Cyanosis** It is common practice to administer oxygen in a concentration just sufficient to relieve cyanosis, while awaiting the results of blood gas measurements.

B. THERAPEUTIC GOALS

1. Maintain Pa_{O_2} in the range of 50 to 100 torr and preferably 60 to 80 torr in small prematures to avoid hypoxia or hyperoxia.

2. When cardiac output and its distribution are normal, oxygen tensions of 40 to 50 torr probably provide for adequate tissue oxygen delivery.

3. In premature infants, oxygen tensions below 50 torr may depress respiratory effort, producing hypoventilation or apneic spells.

4. In near-term and more mature infants, oxygen tensions below 50 torr may significantly increase pulmonary vascular resistance.

5. Under the best of circumstances, it may not be possible to meet your therapeutic goals consistently regarding Pa_{O_2} or F_{IO_2}.

C. MONITORING

The frequency of measurement of arterial oxygen tension is determined by how rapidly the patient's pulmonary status is changing and on the availability of devices for continuously monitoring the status of oxygenation.

1. Infants requiring more than 40% oxygen during the acute phase of their illness should have Pa_{O_2} measurements at least every four hours. More frequent measurements are indicated during the period of instability.

2. Check Pa_{O_2} ten to 30 minutes after making changes in the concentration of oxygen or of ventilator settings.

3. Infants with stable chronic lung disease may only require daily or less frequent determinations.

4. In infants requiring high oxygen concentrations, it is advisable to measure the oxygen tension periodically in the descending aorta and temporal or right radial artery simultaneously. Right-to-left ductal shunts may produce higher Pa_{O_2} values above the ductus than are measured in the descending aorta (umbilical artery catheter).

5. Continuous monitoring of oxygen tension with transcutaneous or intravascular oxygen electrodes is an important advance that improves our ability to maintain blood oxygen tensions in the desired range. This form of monitoring can be useful whenever the devices are available and the personnel understand their use and the interpretation of the information provided.

D. OXYGEN DELIVERY

1. Mixtures of oxygen and air may be delivered to an infant by means of endotracheal tubes, nasal prongs, or tubes, masks,

funnels, and hoods. In general, an oxygen blender should be used with these techniques. Usually, 100% oxygen is administered via nasal cannulae or incubator flooding and the liter flow is adjusted to achieve the desired concentration of oxygen.

2. Warmed, humidified gas should be used whenever possible.

3. The gas flow used may be dependent on the operation requirements of the mixing device, or blender.

   a. Head hood: A liter flow three times the volume of the head hood, or about 6 to 8 L/min, is usually adequate to prevent rebreathing of exhaled carbon dioxide. Higher flows may be necessary to assure stable oxygen concentrations.

   b. Intubated patients: Gas flows one to two times greater than the estimated minute ventilation are adequate in continuous flow systems with a reservoir to provide for the peak inspiratory flow demand. Higher flows may be necessary to achieve the desired level of CPAP.

4. The oxygen concentration delivered to the infant should be routinely measured every hour, or following changes in oxygen delivery, with a recently calibrated oxygen analyzer. If the baby is in an oxygen hood, gas should be sampled near the nose.

E. SPECIAL CONSIDERATIONS

1. Retrolental Fibroplasia (RLF)

   a. Risk increases with decreasing gestational age.

   b. Risk increases with prolonged administration of oxygen.

   c. The duration and magnitude of oxygen exposure required to produce RLF are currently not known.

   d. Other factors, including individual susceptibility and hypercarbia, appear to be important.

   e. Most cases of RLF resolve; however, a few progress to visual impairment, including blindness.

   f. RLF is not totally preventable at present.

   g. Compulsive attention to oxygen therapy may reduce the incidence of RLF, and this is an important goal.

   h. RLF is also known as retinopathy of prematurity.

2. Pulmonary Oxygen Toxicity

a. Often called bronchopulmonary dysplasia (BPD) or chronic lung disease of prematurity (CLD).

b. Most frequently observed in mechanically ventilated infants with prolonged exposure to high oxygen concentrations.

c. Other factors such as lung trauma from the ventilator, individual susceptibility, and preexisting lung disease are probably involved.

d. Efforts to reduce incidence or severity of CLD are currently focused on limiting barotrauma and O_2 exposure.

39

Endotracheal Intubation

A. INDICATIONS

1. In the Delivery Room

a. Severe cardiorespiratory depression (e.g., Apgar 0, 1, or 2).

b. Bag and mask ventilation is unsuccessful.

c. Upper airway obstruction (e.g., Pierre-Robin).

d. Gastrointestinal dilation is undesirable (e.g., suspected diaphragmatic hernia, abdominal wall defect).

e. When meconium aspiration is suspected.

2. In the Intensive Care Nursery

a. Assisted ventilation (mechanical or manual).

b. Therapy with CPAP.

c. Treatment of upper airway obstruction.

d. Tracheobronchial toilet.

e. Tracheal aspiration for microbiologic studies.

B. ROUTE

We routinely use orotracheal intubation because of the relative ease in developing and maintaining proficiency with the technique. On occasion nasotracheal intubation may be desired.

C. ENDOTRACHEAL TUBE

1. We use soft tubes that have markings at 1-cm intervals and a heavy black circumferential line 1.5 or 2 cm from the tip.

2. Tubes may be made stiffer for intubation by using a sterile pipe clearner as a stylet. BE CERTAIN that the stylet ends 2 to 3 mm above the tip of the tube and does not protrude at the side hole.

3. The tube size should allow a small air leak around it.

Patient Weight (gm)	Tube Size (mm)
<1,000	2.5
1,000–2,500	3.0
>2,500	3.5

D. LARYNGOSCOPY

Use a Miller "0" laryngoscope blade for premature infants and a Miller "1" laryngoscope blade for full-term infants. Note: the laryngoscope is a left-handed, lifting instrument.

E. TECHNIQUE

1. Check laryngoscope, suction setup, oxygen and ventilatory equipment before proceeding. Empty the infant's stomach with an orogastric tube.

2. Use clean technique.

3. If the procedure is elective, ventilate the infant with bag and mask and supplemental oxygen for one minute or longer before intubation. Do not bag and mask infants with meconium staining, suspected diaphragmatic hernia, or severe upper airway obstruction. Proceed directly to intubation (Fig. 39–1).

4. Position the patient in "sniff position" with the head slightly extended. Do NOT hyperextend. Suction mucous from the airway under direct vision if needed.

5. Advance the laryngoscope with the left hand, beginning at the right corner of the patient's mouth, rotating to the midline and moving the tongue to the left. When the blade tip is in the space between the tongue and epiglottis, the epiglottis will lift, exposing the glottis and vocal cords.

6. Advance the endotracheal tube along the right side of the

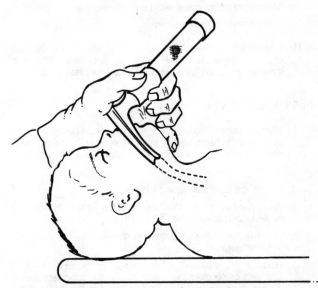

Fig 39–1.—Technique of endotracheal intubation. Note position of hand on laryngoscope handle. (From Goetzmann B.W.: Resuscitation of the newborn, in Niswander K.R. (ed.): Manual of Obstetrics. Boston, Little, Brown & Co., 1980, pp. 389–397. Used by permission.)

laryngoscope blade, but NOT within its C-shaped opening or your line of sight to the glottis will be obstructed.

7. Insert the tip of the tube into the glottis, between the vocal cords, and advance until the black line on the tube is just visible above the cords.

8. For temporary fixation, grasp the endotracheal tube near the mouth with the thumb and finger of the right hand and rest the remainder of the fingers on the infant's cheek.

9. Remove the stylet, attach the ventilating device, and begin manual ventilation with oxygen-enriched gas. If intubation is successful, the following should be present:

 a. A good heart rate response.

b. Movement of the chest with positive-pressure ventilation.

c. Good breath sounds bilaterally.

10. If you cannot insert the endotracheal tube within 30 seconds, ventilate the infant using bag and mask for two to three minutes and try again when the heart rate is stable.

F. TUBE FIXATION

1. After successful intubation, hold the tube securely in place by resting the hand holding the tube against the baby's face. Note the number on the side of the tube at the maxillary gum margin.

2. Secure the tube with tape as follows:

a. Apply benzoin above and below the lips, to the cheeks, and to the endotracheal tube. Allow it to dry.

b. Three-eighth-inch white adhesive tape is cut either in "H" or "Y" configuration.

c. When a "Y" is used, the base is applied to the cheek with one arm going over the lower lip and the other arm going around the endotracheal tube positioned at the corner of the mouth. A second "Y" is applied with the base on the cheek, one arm on the upper lip, and the other arm around the tube in the opposite direction of the first tape.

3. Always check tube position by x-ray and adjust as necessary. The tube should be approximately 1 cm above the carina when the neck is in a neutral position.

G. TUBE REPLACEMENT

Endotracheal tubes need to be changed only if occluded by secretions, when there is accidental dislodgement, or if another diameter is deemed more appropriate.

H. ENDOTRACHEAL TUBE SUCTIONING

This is a sterile procedure; use good technique and powder-free gloves. Isotonic saline, 0.5 ml, should be instilled into the tube prior to suctioning. Suctioning is usually performed every two to three hours. More or less frequent suctioning may be required depending on the amount of secretions and the infant's tolerance to the procedure.

I. ENDOTRACHEAL TUBE REMOVAL

1. Suction the endotracheal tube and ventilate manually for one to two minutes.

2. Suction the oropharynx and empty the stomach.

3. Deftly withdraw the tube during manual inflation of the lungs.

4. Place the infant in an oxygen enriched environment 5% to 10% higher than that delivered via the endotracheal tube. Obtain a blood gas valve in 15 to 30 minutes or follow with transcutaneous Po_2 monitoring.

5. If the tube was in place for one hour or more, maintain the infant NPO for four to eight hours to allow return of glottic closure mechanisms.

6. We do not routinely use dexamethasone or racemic epinephrine, before and after extubation, respectively. On occasion, when extubation has not been successful, these agents are utilized. Consult the attending neonatologist.

7. Observe postextubation stridor and chest wall retractions. Evaluate with arterial blood gas studies and chest x-ray film.

J. COMPLICATIONS

1. Laryngeal trauma, including hematoma and perforation.

2. Vocal cord paralysis.

3. Infection.

4. Subglottic stenosis occurs in 1% to 5% of intubated infants. On occasion, the stenosis will be so severe as to require tracheostomy.

40

Continuous Positive Airway Pressure

A. INTRODUCTION

Continuous positive airway pressure (CPAP), or constant distending airway pressure (CDAP), is useful in improving oxygenation in infants whose lung disease is complicated by loss of lung volume (RDS, pulmonary edema, and diffuse atelectasis). The presumed explanation for its effectiveness is prevention of alveolar collapse during expiration. Many larger infants with RDS can be managed with CPAP alone, while only a small percentage of infants weighing less than 1,500 gm can be carried through their course entirely on CPAP.

B. TECHNIQUES

1. **A Modified Gregory Apparatus** (Fig. 40–1) can be used with the following:

   a. An endotracheal tube

   b. Nasal prongs

   c. A nasopharyngeal catheter or tube

2. **Continuous Negative Pressure (CNP)** (Isolette® negative-pressure ventilator)

C. CPAP PROCEDURE

1. Connect CPAP device, with appropriate gas flow and oxygen concentration, to a properly placed endotracheal tube, nasopharyngeal tube, or nasal prongs.

2. Adjust pressure to 4 to 6 cm water and measure Pa_{O_2} in 15 minutes, or observe response on transcutaneous Po_2 monitor.

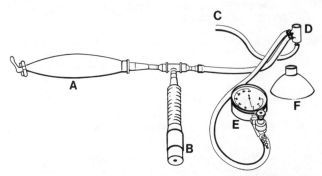

Fig 40-1.—Ventilating device for infant resuscitation. A, *500-ml anesthesia bag;* B, *pressure release valve;* C, *oxygen line;* D, *head (accepts mask or endotracheal tube);* E, *pressure manometer;* F, *infant ventilating mask.* (From Goetzman B.W.: Resuscitation of the newborn, in Niswander K.R. (ed.): Manual of Obstetrics. *Boston, Little, Brown & Co., 1980, pp. 389–397. Used by permission.)*

3. Increase applied pressure by 2-cm water increments until Pa_{O_2} rises above 60 to 70 torr. Usually, we do not exceed 12-cm water. If CPAP fails to increase the Pa_{O_2} above 50 torr, mechanical ventilation is indicated.

4. When the Pa_{O_2} response has been confirmed, begin lowering the inspired oxygen concentration in 5% increments to obtain a Pa_{O_2} between 50 and 80 torr.

5. When the inspired oxygen concentration has been lowered to 40%, decrease the airway pressure in 1-cm water increments. Follow each change with measurement of Pa_{O_2} in 15 to 20 minutes unless response is being observed on a transcutaneous Po_2 monitor. Usually, a change is made at two-hour intervals unless the Pao_2 is greater than 100 torr. More rapid changes are then indicated to lower the Pa_{O_2} below 100 torr.

6. When an applied pressure to 2 to 3 cm water is tolerated for four hours or more, the infant may be extubated and placed in a head hood with an inspired oxygen concentration 5% to 10% higher than that used on CPAP. Reassess Pa_{O_2} and Pa_{CO_2} in 15 to 20 minutes.

7. While undergoing CPAP, most infants are ventilated manually or sighed for three to five minutes every 30 to 60 minutes during the acute phase, and every three to four hours during

resolution. This may be continued, by bag and mask, for 24 hours following extubation.

8. Most infants requiring assisted ventilation with positive end-expiratory pressure are subsequently changed to CPAP therapy, and the procedures outlined in 5 through 7 above are then followed prior to extubation.

9. Infants weighing less than 1,250 gm frequently do not tolerate CPAP during the preextubation period, but may be successfully extubated from low pressure ventilation.

D. CONTINUOUS NEGATIVE PRESSURE

The infant is placed in a chamber (Isolette® negative-pressure ventilator) with his head outside the chamber. The chamber is sealed at the neck with an iris diaphragm. Negative pressure (partial vacuum) is then developed around the body and a constant distending airway pressure is developed that is identical in action to CPAP. Oxygen mixtures are delivered to the infant by hood or funnel. The procedure for instituting and withdrawing CNP is the same as for CPAP except that pressure changes are negative-pressure increments around the body.

E. COMPLICATIONS

1. Pneumothorax occurs in about 15% of infants so treated.

2. When applied to normal lungs or at high pressure levels in abnormal lungs, decreased venous return with decreased cardiac output, tamponade of pulmonary capillaries, and decreased ventilation have been observed.

41

Chest Physiotherapy: Percussion, Vibration and Suctioning

A. PURPOSE

The purpose of percussion, vibration, and suctioning (PVS) therapy is to improve the clearance of mucous and debris from the airways. These techniques are often fatiguing to the infant and time consuming for the nurse and therefore need to be used judiciously.

B. INDICATIONS AND FREQUENCY

1. The use of PVS is indicated in patients with pulmonary secretions and prophylactically in patients with chronic lung disease and impaired respiratory movement (e.g., paralyzed infants).

2. **Frequency** depends on productivity of secretions, therapeutic goals, and tolerance.

   a. PVS orders must be individualized, not ritualized, and frequently reassessed.

   b. Personnel providing PVS therapy are often the best judges of productivity and tolerance. If a baby fights PVS, particularly during bagging, blood gases may deteriorate for up to 30 minutes.

   c. Patient tolerance of PVS therapy should be evaluated initially and periodically using a transcutaneous oxygen monitor. Patients who have cardiorespiratory instability are the most likely to deteriorate during the procedure.

3. **General Guidelines for PVS Orders**

   a. *RDS:* The acute phase (first 48 hours) is not accompanied by significant tracheobronchial secretions, and PVS is usually not needed. Routine endotracheal suctioning should suffice. At about 48 hours of age, an exudative phase begins and PVS on a three- to four-hour basis (usually before feedings) is helpful. As the RDS resolves, the frequency of PVS can be decreased.

b. *Meconium aspiration:* PVS at two to four hours may be helpful during the first 8 to 12 hours of age. After that a lesser frequency should suffice.

c. *Pneumonia:* PVS is usually of benefit when there are increased secretions.

d. *Atelectasis of Isolated Lobes:* PVS may be limited to those areas.

e. *Paralyzed and comatose infants* and infants with chronic lung disease probably benefit from a routine PVS every eight to 12 hours whether or not secretions are evident. However, benefit from a routine long-term prophylactic PVS must be reevaluated periodically.

42

Ventilatory Assistance

I. BAG AND MASK VENTILATION

Ventilation by bag and mask is easily learned and is usually an effective means of establishing lung expansion. Its success rate is usually only limited by the availability of an appropriate size mask and the experience of the operator.

A. INDICATIONS

1. Used in resuscitation and in managing infants for short periods of time while preparing for intubation.

2. Precautions in the Delivery Room

   a. Infants suspected of meconium aspiration should be intubated and suctioned before positive-pressure ventilation is used.

   b. Bag and mask ventilation should not be used if a diaphragmatic hernia is suspected.

   c. Very small infants and infants with micrognathia usually cannot be ventilated effectively by bag and mask, and immediate intubation may be necessary. With severe micrognathia and airway obstruction (Pierre-Robin anomaly), ventilation may be possible through a nasopharyngeal tube (an endotracheal tube passed through the nose and past the tongue obstruction).

3. Used intermittently to treat or prevent postextubation atelectasis.

B. EQUIPMENT

We usually use an anesthesia bag and mask with an attached pressure manometer. An Ohio self-inflating infant resuscitator with the accumulator attached to permit delivery of a high F_{IO_2} is also satisfactory.

C. TECHNIQUE

1. Mask is held firmly over the face with the head in neutral position and finger lifting chin. Mask should not rest on eye.

2. Usual respiratory frequency is 30 to 50 per minute.

3. Usual inspiratory pressure is 20 to 30 cm water.

4. Pressures of 30 to 60 cm of H_2O are occasionally required during initial resuscitation in the delivery room.

D. ASSESSMENT

1. In the delivery room, a return of a normal heart rate and absence of central cyanosis usually indicates adequate O_2 delivery.

2. One should be able to observe chest expansion and auscultate good air entry bilaterally when effective ventilation is provided.

3. Frequent monitoring by arterial blood gas volumes is required in prolonged resuscitation.

E. COMPLICATIONS

1. **Pneumothorax**

2. **Gaseous Distention of Stomach** may require orogastric tube or discontinuing enteral feedings.

3. **Patient Fatigue** with subsequent hypoventilation, apneic spells, or both.

4. **Abrasions of Facial Skin**

5. **Retinal Detachment** Keep mask off eyes and do not use excessive pressure to apply mask.

6. **REMEMBER** Intermittent bag and mask may worsen blood gases if the baby fights the procedure. It is necessary to evaluate each patient's response to therapy.

II. MECHANICAL VENTILATION

The hallmark of the newborn intensive care unit is the ability to manage long-term assisted ventilation of sick newborns successfully. Styles of ventilation (rapid vs. slow, long vs. short inspiratory times, etc.) may differ among institutions. Many styles have proven effective. A uniform team approach (physician, nurse, respiratory therapist, radiologist, and clinical laboratory) is essential. The brand of equipment used is not critical. Success is determined by how well you use the equipment you have.

A. INDICATIONS

Respiratory failure may occur in infants with a wide range of disorders, including lung disease heart disease, intrathoracic anomalies, CNS depression by drugs or disease, and in premature infants with severe apneic spells. When respiratory failure is severe and other methods for treating pulmonary insufficiency have failed, mechanical ventilation is indicated.

B. EQUIPMENT

We use the Baby Bird®, Sechrist®, or other pressure-limited infant ventilators. On occasion we use the Isolette® negative-pressure ventilator for long-term ventilatory assistance of large babies.

C. PRINCIPLES OF THERAPY

1. Techniques available for improving oxygenation in noncompliant lungs include the following:

   a. Increased concentration of inspired oxygen

   b. Increased inspiratory pressure

   c. Increased positive end-expiratory pressure (PEEP)

   d. Increased inspiratory time (I:E ratio)

   e. Inspiratory pressure plateau (square pressure wave)

2. Techniques available for improving ventilation (carbon dioxide removal) include the following:

   a. Increased tidal volume

   b. Increased rate

   c. Prolonging the expiratory time (in some circumstances)

3. Ventilator settings (rate, inspiratory pressure, inspiratory pressure plateau, I:E ratio, and PEEP) will vary depending on the pathologic entity involved and on the measured response to a particular therapeutic trial.

D. GOALS

1. Smoothly regulate the Pa_{O_2} in a range of 50 to 100 torr.

2. Avoid hypoxia (Pa_{O_2} <50 torr) and hyperoxia (Pa_{O_2} >100 torr).

3. Maintain the Pa_{CO_2} in the range of 35 to 45 torr.

4. Certain conditions may require accepting Pa_{O_2} and Pa_{CO_2} limits other than those given above.

   a. In chronic lung disease, a higher Pa_{CO_2} may be acceptable.

   b. In cyanotic heart disease, a lower Pa_{O_2} may be acceptable.

   c. In pulmonary hypertension, a higher Pa_{O_2} may be acceptable.

5. The decision to intervene with support techniques other than supplemental oxygen should be documented in the chart according to the criteria in section IIA.

E. TECHNIQUE

1. Typical initial ventilator settings in RDS are as follows:

   a. Inspiratory pressure of 20 to 24 cm of water.

   b. PEEP of 4 to 6 cm of water.

   c. Frequency of 20 to 24 per minute.

   d. Inspiratory time of 0.4 to 0.8 seconds.

2. In an infant with normal lungs and severe apneic spells, the initial settings might be as follows:

    a. Inspiratory pressure of 14 to 16 cm water.

    b. PEEP of 2 to 4 cm water.

    c. Rate of 15–20 per minute.

3. Manipulation of flow and inspiratory time controls on the Baby Bird and of the wave form control on the Sechrist may allow the pressure wave form to be altered.

4. Remember, the ventilator cycles automatically and is not triggered by the infant. Since there is a continuous flow of fresh gas past the endotracheal tube when the ventilator is in the expiratory phase, the infant will establish its own respiratory rate, usually two to four times the frequency of the ventilator.

5. A well-ventilated infant usually gets in phase with the ventilator cycling, unless he is disturbed. If he is agitated this may impair the effectiveness of the ventilator and medication.

    a. Morphine sulfate, 0.1 mg/kg, may be used as a sedative.

    b. Sometimes an infant may fight the ventilator to such an extent that paralysis is indicated. Pancuronium bromide, 0.06 to 0.10 mg/kg, is the recommended drug for this purpose. Consult the neonatal fellow or attending physician concerning paralysis. Remember, a paralyzed or heavily sedated infant loses his ability to breathe and will require a higher ventilator rate. In addition, he must be CONSTANTLY observed for accidental extubation or mechanical failure of the ventilator.

F. ASSESSMENT

1. Effective ventilation involves a continuous series of trial and error manipulations. Frequent reevaluation of the total patient, including blood gas volumes, is essential. Each patient is unique in his or her response to ventilator changes.

2. One should be able to observe chest expansion and auscultate good air entry bilaterally when effective ventilation is provided.

3. A well-oxygenated and ventilated patient is usually well perfused, centrally acyanotic, and comfortable.

G. COMPLICATIONS

1. **Alveolar Rupture** with formation of pulmonary interstitial emphysema, pneumothorax, or pneumomediastinum is the most common complication of mechanical ventilation. This occurs in about 20% of RDS infants requiring mechanical ventilation in our nursery.

2. **Other Complications** include the following:

    a. Bacterial colonization and infection

    b. Obstructed endotracheal tube or extubation

    c. Intubation of the right main-stem bronchus

    d. Pneumopericardium with cardiac tamponade

    e. Impaired venous return and decreased cardiac output

    f. Chronic lung disease

    g. Stenosis and obstruction of the trachea

H. WITHDRAWAL OF VENTILATORY SUPPORT

1. Withdrawal of ventilatory support is a technique for testing the infant to see how well he manages without the ventilator. The process has often been referred to as "weaning." This is a poor term because it implies that you may be able to teach the patient to get along without the ventilator.

2. In general, ventilatory support is to be used only in the amounts necessary to provide adequate ventilation and oxygenation. One should always strive to use the minimum support necessary to achieve that goal.

3. Withdrawal of ventilatory support must be individualized. Reduce that parameter which is considered to be most excessive and most hazardous to the patient, as tolerated.

4. When a rate of 10 to 12 respirations per minute is tolerated, the infant can usually be changed to CPAP at 4 to 6 cm water (or to CNP). The inspired oxygen concentration is kept the same or raised by 5%. At this point an arterial blood gas value is obtained in ten to 15 minutes. Some infants who weigh less than 1,250 gm do not tolerate CPAP, but do well if extubated when ventilator settings are low.

5. **CAUTION**   When using slow rates (10 to 15 respirations per minute), avoid excessive inspiratory times. An inspiratory time of 0.5 seconds should be adequate and certainly should not exceed 1.0 seconds. Thus, at a rate of 15 respirations per minute the I:E ratio should be 1:3-10. Remember, slowing the rate by increasing the inspiratory time increases mean airway pressure. When ordering a rate change, be sure to specify a change in inspiratory time, expiration time, or both. Be specific in your orders.

6. If at any point during the above process the infant's blood gas status falls into an unacceptable range, immediately return to the previously effective ventilator settings. Reassess the infant for complications of ventilatory therapy for a possible new problem such as patent ductus arteriosus, low hematocrit reading, cold stress, atelectasis, mechanical problem with the ventilatory system, etc.

43

Thoracostomy Drainage
for Pneumothorax

A. NEEDLE THORACOSTOMY

1. Indications

  a. Nontension pneumothorax on chest x-ray film causing significant respiratory compromise.

  b. Confirmed tension pneumothorax.

  c. Sudden life-threatening deterioration in blood gas volume without x-ray confirmation when tension pneumothorax is suspected.

2. Technique

  a. Twenty-gauge (or smaller) short-bevel needles are recommended.

  b. Use a quick, betadine preparation and advance the needle into the intrapleural space via the third intercostal space at the midclavicular line or just anterior to the anterior axillary line. Avoid the areola and nipple.

  c. Gently aspirate air and confirm results roentgenographically.

B. CHEST TUBE PLACEMENT

1. Indications Satisfactory decompression of a tension pneumothorax usually requires continuous suction via a chest tube connected to an underwater seal. Aspiration with a needle and syringe usually gives temporary relief in infants requiring assisted ventilation, but may be all that is required in infants who are breathing spontaneously.

2. Technique

a. Prepare with betadine and alcohol, drape area, wear sterile gloves, and pass instruments in a sterile fashion.

b. The site of insertion may be in the second to fourth intercostal space just below the midclavicular line (preferred) or in the fourth to sixth intercostal space in the anterior axillary line.

c. A red Robinson catheter (size 10-18 French) is preferred. The use of trocar catheters (size 12 French) may cause pulmonary lacerations.

d. Add one or two side holes about 1 cm above the precut hole. Make ½-cm skin incision with a No. 15 scalpel blade. Make a tract with a closed, curved Kelly forceps, allowing air to leak. Either grasp the tube between the blades of the forceps or place the closed tip of the forceps into the tip of the catheter via the first side hole. Advance the catheter along the tract into the pleural space, directing the catheter across the anterior thorax. Remove the forceps and advance the catheter 1 to 2 cm past the last side hole.

e. Connect the chest tube either to a chest-tube suction apparatus at 10 cm water, or on occasion to a Heimlich valve (e.g., during transport of an infant).

f. Anchor chest tubes securely with a purse-string suture (4-0 silk) and a high-tie. Cover site with bacitracin ointment and a small dressing.

g. Obtain an arterial blood gas volume, BP measurement, and chest x-ray film immediately after placing the tube to assess the effectiveness of the tube and its position.

C. CHEST TUBE REMOVAL

1. Indications

a. Pulmonary air leak has sealed, as indicated by cessation of bubbling from the chest tube for 24 hours.

b. Pneumothorax has disappeared on roentgenographic inspection.

c. Pneumothorax does not reappear after four hours' clamping of the chest tube or cessation of bubbling for at least four to six hours on water seal.

2. Technique

   a. At the end of the inspiration phase, rapidly remove the tube while covering the wound with a small sterile dressing holding a "dab" of betadine ointment to produce an airtight seal.

   b. The wound may then be closed with a 4-0 silk suture.

   c. Follow the infant's vital signs closely and obtain a follow-up chest x-ray film.

44

Pericardiocentesis for Pneumopericardium

A. INDICATIONS

1. Pericardial air, on chest x-ray film, causing cardiovascular compromise.

2. Sudden, life-threatening deterioration in blood gases and circulation without x-ray confirmation when cardiac tamponade is suspected; transillumination may be helpful in locating air collection.

3. Tamponade secondary to fluid or blood collection.

B. TECHNIQUE

1. A 20-gauge angiocatheter or a 19 to 22-gauge intracatheter, T-tube connection, three-way stopcock, and sterile syringe are needed.

2. The subxyphoid area is prepped with betadine.

3. The angiocatheter is advanced from the subxyphoid position toward left midclavicle at about a 30° angle with the chest wall. Once a "pop" is sensed, negative pressure is applied to the syringe to aspirate air or other contents. The catheter is then advanced and sewn in place with the T-tube connector attached to an underwater seal at -10 cm H_2O pressure.

4. Alternatively, an intracatheter with one or two additional side holes is used. An ECG is connected with precordial lead attached to the intracatheter needle via a double alligator clip. The ECG is set to record in the precordial position. A tracing is present when the skin is contacted, disappears when the needle is advanced subcutaneously, and reappears when the pericardium is entered. The catheter is then advanced, secured, and attached as above.

45

Blood Sampling Techniques

A. HEEL STICKS

1. **Purpose** To obtain small amounts (1 ml or less) of blood.

2. **Technique**
   a. The large lancets, in red envelopes, are used for larger premature and term infants. The small lancets, in blue envelopes, are used exclusively for small premature infants.
   b. Insert the lancet in the posterior lateral instep.

B. ARTERIAL PUNCTURES

1. **Purpose** To obtain blood for arterial blood gas analysis. Radial and temporal arteries are the most accessible and are safest for percutaneous arterial sampling. Radial artery puncture is described in detail.

2. **Equipment** The same equipment is used for each site and is of individual preference.
   a. Heparinized tuberculin syringe with a 25-gauge needle, or
   b. 25-gauge butterfly preflushed with heparin and connected to a syringe by assistant after blood flow has been established.

3. **Technique**
   a. Feel radial artery pulse and enter skin just above the proximal wrist crease and about one sixth the distance across the wrist.
   b. Advance the needle (level up) at a 45° angle, penetrating the artery.
   c. Slowly withdraw the needle until blood returns.

C. UMBILICAL ARTERIAL CATHETERS

1. Equipment

a. Sampling syringes

b. Flush syringes

2. Procedure

a. Place the stopcock and tubing on a sterile pad.

b. Clean the stopcock with an alcohol sponge.

c. For ABG and usual laboratory studies, clear the line by withdrawing 2 to 3 cc of blood. For coagulation studies, clear the line by withdrawing 4 cc of blood. DO NOT obtain samples for blood glucose determinations from an indwelling catheter.

d. Disconnect the syringe, letting one drop of blood overflow. For arterial blood gas, draw 0.3 ml of blood into heparinized TB syringe, expel air, attach stopper, and place on ice.

e. Reinfuse the 2 to 3 ml of blood previously withdrawn and clear the line with 0.5 ml normal saline.

f. Chart volumes of blood removed and saline infused.

46

Placement and Management
of Intravascular Catheters

I. UMBILICAL ARTERIAL CATHETER

A. INDICATIONS

1. Arterial Blood Gas Monitoring

a. Anticipating a need for more than four samples per day for more than two days.

b. Inspired oxygen requirement greater than 40%.

2. Arterial Blood Pressure Monitoring

B. PERMISSIBLE USES (NOT INDICATIONS)

1. Fluid, glucose, and electrolyte administrations. All infusates should contain heparin, 0.5 to 1.0 units per milliliter.

2. Antibiotic administration (if other site is not available).

3. Drawing blood specimens.

4. Blood transfusion and blood product infusion.

5. Exchange transfusion.

6. Alkali therapy.

C. PROHIBITED SUBSTANCES (EXCEPT IN RESUSCITATION)

1. Infusion of concentrated calcium solutions of 400 to 600 mg/dl.

2. Tolazoline.

3. Parenteral nutrition solutions (except with attending physician's approval).

4. Glucose concentrations in excess of 12.5%, excluding TPN.

5. Known vasotoxic drugs.

D. INDICATIONS FOR REMOVAL

1. Thromboembolic complications.

2. When FIO_2 is below 0.30 to 0.40.

E. EQUIPMENT REQUIRED

1. Sterilized umbilical artery catheterization trays supplemented with the following:
   a. Argyle umbilical artery catheter (UAC)—No. 3.5 French for infants with birth weight under 1,500 gm, No. 5 French for larger infants.
   b. Three-way stockcock attached to a blunt needle.
   c. Umbilical tape.
   d. Scalpel blade.

F. INSERTION OF UAC

1. Attach the infant to a cardiac monitor. Sterile gloves, clean gown, mask, and cap must be worn by the operator. Prepare the cord and surrounding skin thoroughly with betadine while a nurse holds the cord suspended. Drape the infant, but allow for observation.

2. Place umbilical tape loosely around the umbilical stump (to be used for hemorrhage control). Cut the umbilical cord 1 to 2 cm from skin with a scalpel (not scissors) and drape.

3. Grasp cord with thumb forceps and hold upright. When the cut surface is blotted, the umbilical vessels can be identified: the single, large, thin-walled oval vein can readily be distinguished from the two smaller, thick-walled, round arteries.

4. The closed tips of the small curved iris forceps should be gently inserted into the lumen of one artery until the cut end of the artery is at the bend in the forceps; the spring of the forceps is allowed to spread the tips apart, thus dilating the artery. Repeatedly dilate the lumen until the orifice appears large enough to accommodate the catheter.

5. Grasp the catheter about 1 cm from the tip between the thumb and forefinger or with forceps, and while the cord stump is held upright, insert the catheter into the lumen of the dilated artery. An assistant may grasp the arterial wall with forceps to facilitate insertion of the catheter. The catheter may encounter obstruction at the level of the anterior abdominal wall or the bladder. Obstruction can usually be overcome within 60 seconds (by the clock) of gentle, steady pressure. Don't attempt to force the catheter. As a last resort, remove the catheter, empty the saline, partially fill with 2% xylocaine without epinephrine, fill with normal saline so that xylocaine now fills tip of catheter, reinsert catheter, and infuse 0.1 to 0.2 ml of xylocaine. Wait one to two minutes until the drug has relaxed the vasospasm, then advance the catheter.

6. If unsuccessful, catheterization of the other artery should be attempted. If difficulty is encountered, consult fellow or attending physician. Catheter tip should lie at L3–4 and ALWAYS be verified by an abdominal x-ray film.

G. STABILIZATION OF CATHETER

1. When the catheter has been inserted to the desired length, ensure that there is free flow of blood before the catheter is stabilized.

2. Flush the catheters. Observe both legs for evidence of blanching, cyanosis, or mottling.

3. Place a purse-string suture in the interior wall of the cord *around* the catheter. Tie the suture snugly, but not so tightly that you kink the catheter. Leave the ends of the suture long. Wrap these around the catheter about 0.5 cm from the end of the cord using a clove hitch and then tie with a square knot.

4. Paint the abdomen with tincture of benzoin and allow to dry. Secure catheter to a tape bridge.

5. Apply antibiotic ointment to umbilicus stump.

6. Attach catheter and stopcock to IV tubing, making sure all bubbles have been removed from the system. Begin infusion to prevent blood from clotting in the catheter.

H. REMOVAL OF CATHETER

1. Cut and remove sutures holding catheter in place.

2. Gently loosen adhesive tape from skin.

3. Withdraw catheter and apply pressure with 2×2 sponges. Maintenance of pressure for up to five minutes is usually adequate to stop bleeding. Insertion of a purse-string suture may be necessary if bleeding continues.

4. Apply antibiotic ointment to the umbilicus.

5. Observe umbilicus for bleeding.

II. RADIAL ARTERY CATHETERS

A. INDICATIONS

1. Arterial blood gas monitoring

2. Arterial blood pressure monitoring

3. When UAC placement is not possible, a UAC thromboembolic complication has occurred or surgery requires ABG and blood pressure monitoring.

B. PERMISSIBLE USES (NOT INDICATIONS)

1. Fluid administration

2. Sodium administration (0.2 or 0.25 normal sodium chloride in 5% dextrose in water containing 0.5 to 1.0 units of heparin per milliliter of infusate to maintain catheter patency).

3. Drawing blood specimens

C. PROHIBITED SUBSTANCES Known vasotoxic substances.

D. EQUIPMENT

1. Medicine needle, 22 gauge

2. Short extension tubing, T-tube

E. TECHNIQUE

1. Occlude radial artery by compression for 30 seconds to ensure adequate collateral circulation to the hand (modified Allen test).

2. Fix arm-to-arm board with wrist in slight extension. Do not obstruct view of fingers.

3. Percutaneous radial artery catheter (same as arterial puncture).

   a. Identify radial artery pulse.

   b. Insert needle at 30° to 40° angle from forearm for a distance of 0.5 to 1.0 cm.

   c. Remove needle and slowly withdraw catheter until blood returns. Then angle catheter slightly and advance until resistance is met.

   d. Attach extension tubing, withdraw arterial blood gas sample, and slowly flush with heparinized saline.

   e. Fix the catheter in place with tape and secure extension tubing.

4. Radial artery cutdown

   a. If unsuccessful with percutaneous catheter, let vessel recover for one hour (if possible) before proceeding.

   b. Identify location of radial artery pulse and surgically prepare area. Use sterile surgical technique.

   c. Anesthetize locally with 1% lidocaine and make superficial 0.5- to 1.0-cm skin incision across wrist medial to the radial styloid process (at or just above the proximal wrist crease).

   d. Carefully blunt dissect tissue, identifying the radial artery (it may not pulsate visibly).

e. Puncture the vessel, inserting the Medicut® (or similar catheter) at a 30° angle (from the wrist-forearm) through the artery.

f. Remove the needle and gently remove the catheter until the tip is in the lumen. Blood flow usually returns unless the artery is in spasm. Then advance the catheter until resistance is met.

g. DO NOT ligate the radial artery or tie suture around the vessel and catheter. The vessel will recanalize following removal.

h. When blood returns, attach the extension tubing and flush the catheter slowly with heparinized saline.

i. Stabilize the catheter with tape and sutures used in wound closure.

F. INDICATIONS FOR REMOVAL

1. Inflammation or thromboembolic complications

2. When no longer needed.

III. UMBILICAL VENOUS CATHETER (UVC)

A. INDICATIONS

1. Central venous pressure monitoring

2. Exchange transfusion

3. Resuscitation

B. PERMISSIBLE USES (NOT INDICATIONS)

1. Fluid, glucose, and electrolyte administration

2. Alkali therapy

3. Antibiotic therapy

4. Blood product or albumin infusions

5. Drawing blood specimens

C. PROHIBITED SUBSTANCES

1. Parenteral nutrition solutions

2. Known cardiotoxic drugs

D. INDICATIONS FOR REMOVAL   Catheter should be removed within 48 hours unless critically needed.

E. PLACEMENT TECHNIQUE

1. Cut umbilical stump 1 to 2 cm from skin.

2. Grasp umbilicus with thumb forceps and gently probe vein lumen. Since the vein extends cephalad from the umbilicus, the entering probe may be held almost parallel to the abdomen below the umbilicus. Remove any visible clots with a forceps.

3. Ensure that the catheter is filled with saline and attached to a syringe when it is introduced. Extreme care must be taken that the catheter is not open to the atmosphere, since air embolus can occur if the infant takes a deep inspiration producing a negative pressure in the thoracic inferior vena cava.

4. Verify location of the catheter tip by x-ray film or venous pressure tracing. If the tip is in the liver, slowly remove the catheter until blood can no longer be withdrawn and then advance to 0.5 cm. This will prevent infusing hypertonic or toxic substances directly into the lower hepatic circulation.

IV. PERCUTANEOUS PERIPHERAL VENOUS CATHETER

A. INDICATIONS

1. Intravenous line for critical period or surgery

2. Intravenous line when scalp veins are not available

B. PERMISSIBLE USES

1. Fluid, glucose, and electrolyte administration

2. Blood or albumin infusions

3. Antibiotic therapy

C. DURATION OF CATHETERIZATION

1. Seventy-two hours or less

2. Remove if swelling or inflammation is observed

V. PERCUTANEOUS DEEP VENOUS CATHETER

A. INDICATIONS

1. Intravenous line for parenteral nutrition

2. Intravenous line for fluids and electrolytes

B. PERMISSIBLE USES

1. Parenteral nutrition solutions

2. Closed-system glucose and electrolyte solutions

C. PROHIBITED SUBSTANCES   All drugs and substances that cannot be added in the pharmacy.

D. INDICATIONS FOR REMOVAL

1. Sepsis

2. Occlusion of catheter

3. Vascular complications

4. Adequate oral and peripheral vein nutrition

E. EQUIPMENT

1. Silastic radiopaque medical grade tubing 0.7 mm outside diameter, 0.3 mm inside diameter in 30- and 40-cm lengths.

2. Twenty-seven-gauge blunt needle

3. Nineteen-gauge scalp vein needle

4. Fine forceps

F. PERCUTANEOUS PLACEMENT   An antecubital, external jugular, or scalp vein can be used.

1. For an antecubital vein placement, the extremity is taped on an armboard. A soft rubber band acts as a tourniquet.

2. The skin is cleansed with betadine and draped with sterile towels.

3. The catheter is attached to a 27-gauge blunt needle and flushed with heparinized saline.

4. A 19-gauge scalp-vein needle with the plastic tubing cut off is introduced a short distance into the vein, and using fine forceps, the catheter is threaded into the needle. The catheter is advanced 1 or 2 mm at a time, until it is thought to be in the superior vena cava. When an arm vein is used, the catheter occasionally will meet resistance at the shoulder. Manipulation of the arm often makes it possible to pass this resistance.

5. The scalp-vein needle is then withdrawn, the catheter removed from the blunt needle, and the scalp-vein needle discarded.

6. A 2.5-cm segment of the scalp-vein needle tubing can be inserted over the catheter before it is reattached to the blunt needle to protect the catheter from being punctured by the tip of the blunt needle.

7. Position of the catheter tip in the superior vena cava should be confirmed by x-ray film. Collodion is then applied at the catheter insertion site to prevent slippage.

8. The site is covered with dry gauze or Op-Site.® The blunt needle is connected to a T-connector, which is connected to the IV tubing. A strip of pH paper placed beneath the blunt needle and catheter will identify any leakage of solution.

G. CUTDOWN   Alternatively, a Silastic® catheter can be introduced via a cutdown.

a. The basilic vein in the antecubital fossa is most commonly used.

b. Following preparation of the extremity (as above), the area is infiltrated with 1% lidocaine, and a small incision is made in the medial antecubital fossa.

c. The basilic vein is located by blunt dissection, a ligature placed beneath it, and the vessel nicked with the scalpel; the pointed Silastic catheter, attached to the blunt needle and filled with heparinized saline, is inserted with the fine forceps and advanced into the superior vena cava.

d. The position is confirmed by x-ray film, the wound is sutured, and the site is covered with a dry, sterile gauze or Op-Site.®

47

Continuous Blood Gas Monitoring

Continuous monitoring of pO_2 may be accomplished by a heated Clark skin electrode or a catheter-tip polarographic electrode adapted for an umbilical artery catheter, and pCO_2 can be monitored transcutaneously by a pH-sensitive glass electrode.

A. CATHETER-TIP ELECTRODE

The catheter-tip electrode correlates well with paO_2 and should be considered when placing an umbilical artery catheter in patients in whom rapidly fluctuating paO_2 is anticipated, as in cases of pulmonary hypertension or severe hyaline membrane disease.

B. TRANSCUTANEOUS pO_2 ELECTRODE

1. Principles of Application

a. The skin is maintained at a preset temperature by heated electrode, as shown.
   i. Term infants, 44°C to 45°C.
   ii. Premature infants, 43°C to 44°C.

b. The heat energy required to maintain temperature is a good indicator of relative perfusion to the area.

c. The transcutaneous pO_2 ($TcPO_2$) is not identical to paO_2 and relationship must be established for each patient. Correlation coefficients should be 0.92 or better if properly used.

d. The response time is about 15 to 20 seconds.

2. Indications   Primarily to evaluate episodic variations in pO_2.

a. Prevention of hypoxia or hyperoxia in sick infants

b. Evaluation of effects of nursing procedures on oxygenation, e.g., tracheal tube care, PVS, feeding

c. Evaluation of apnea

d. Monitoring patients during surgery or infant transport

3. Causes of Poor Correlation Between pao_2 and $TcPO_2$

a. Poor skin perfusion
   i. Local ischemia, e.g., skin stretched taut over rib when applying electrode
   ii. Shock or compromised cardiac output

b. Crying while sampling blood by arterial puncture produces a decreased pao_2, which may not be reflected in the cutaneous pao_2 for 20 to 30 seconds.

c. Right-to-left shunting through the ductus arteriosus will produce a higher $TcPO_2$ in the right upper chest than over the abdomen.

d. Inaccurate arterial blood sampling or ABG determination.

4. Complications (Due to Heating Element)

a. Transient erythema may last for several days.

b. Blister formation (uncommon except in small prematures).

C. TRANSCUTANEOUS pco_2 ELECTRODE

1. Principles of Application

a. Utilizes a heated glass pH electrode and a silver reference electrode.

b. Principle of arterialization of cutaneous capillary blood is same as for $TcPO_2$ electrode.

c. Value given on readout must be corrected for diffusion, if correction is not built into the instrument.

d. Response time is about three minutes.

2. Indications   To evaluate episodic variations in pco_2.

a. To evaluate therapy in chronic lung disease.

b. To evaluate respiratory drive response in recurrent apnea or sleep disorders.

c. Evaluation of ventilator therapy.

48

Obtaining Spinal Fluid

The four procedures available for collection of CSF are lumbar, subdural, cisternal, and ventricular punctures.

A. LUMBAR PUNCTURE

1. Lumbar puncture is most frequently used for obtaining CSF for diagnostic purposes. It may be performed in either the lateral recumbent or sitting position. In sick premature infants being ventilated, or with chest tubes inserted, the procedure is more easily done in the lateral recumbent position. The surface on which the infant is placed should be firm and flat. The infant is restrained with hips flexed.

2. Prepare the skin over the lumbar area, as for a surgical procedure.

3. Pertinent landmarks are the spinous processes and iliac crests. The line joining the tops of the iliac crests passes through the fourth spinous process. The space above (3rd) and two spaces below (4th and 5th) are the site of choice for puncture.

4. The needle and obturator are inserted into the chosen vertebral space in the exact midline and perpendicular to the plane of the body. When the dura mater is pierced, remove the obdurator and examine the needle hub for the appearance of fluid.

5. When the fluid is obtained, collect samples in tubes 1, 2, and 3 for the following studies: protein, sugar, cell count, culture and sensitivity, and Gram's stain. Concurrent blood glucose level should be obtained for comparison. "Dry" taps and

bloody taps are more frequent in neonates. However, the presence of blood may be a pathological finding.

B. CISTERNAL, SUBDURAL, AND VENTRICULAR PUNCTURES   are usually performed by the neurosurgery service.

49

Suprapubic Aspiration of Urine

A. INDICATION

1. To obtain a urine specimen for culture and sensitivity in a sick infant in whom the possibility of urinary tract infection exists.

B. EQUIPMENT

1. Antiseptic solution, e.g., betadine

2. Three- to six-milliliter sterile syringe

3. Twenty-two-gauge 1 ½-in needle

C. PROCEDURE

1. Ensure that the patient has not just voided.

2. The infant is placed on a flat surface.

3. An assistant stands opposite the operator and immobilizes the infant by grasping the lower thorax with one hand, and the thighs and hips with the other. Occlusion of the urethra in the male will prevent reflex voiding during cleansing and needle insertion.

4. Operator locates the symphysis pubis with one finger and inserts the needle 1 to 2 cm above the symphysis in the midline and perpendicular to the flat surface.

5. With a single steady motion, the needle is inserted until a perceptible change in resistance is felt as the needle enters the bladder. Light suction is applied to aspirate the urine specimen. It may be necessary to rotate the needle if the bevel is against the bladder wall.

D. COMPLICATIONS

Essentially a benign procedure, the most frequent complication has been transient hematuria. Entering the bowel in a dehydrated patient with resultant fistula formation has been reported.

50

Administration of Blood and Blood Products

A. BLOOD SUPPLY

Since newborns require small volumes of blood (except for exchange transfusions), a single-donor unit of blood can provide multiple transfusions, provided the unit has attached satellite bags. Donor screening techniques are now available to ensure that all blood used for transfusions of newborns is negative for B virus hepatitis and negative for antibodies to CMV.

B. USE OF BLOOD IN THE NURSERY

1. All Rh-positive infants can be transfused with Rh-negative blood if necessary or convenient.

   a. Normally, infants should be given cross-matched, type-specific blood.

   b. For emergencies, group O Rh-negative cells should be requested. Fresh-frozen AB plasma can be requested (for volume expansion or correction for clotting disorders) if required. (Note: cross-match specimens should be taken before transfusions.)

2. Exchange Transfusion

   a. Use modified whole blood that is less than 36 to 48 hours old. It contains viable platelets if it is fresh. Blood for exchanges should always be compatible with the mother's serum specimen so that whole blood can be used if the mother's and the infant's ABO blood group is identical.

   b. A postexchange specimen (contains both infant's and donor's blood) should be sent for future matching against new blood donors. For the second and subsequent exchange transfusions, the donor blood should be cross-matched against both the mother and the infant. If the blood available is more than 48 hours old, it may be necessary to administer platelets.

3. Infants who are premature and only need replacement blood because of frequent blood drawing or from chronic anemia due to prematurity can be transfused with blood that is up to seven days old.

4. A whole or part of a Pedi-pack® set can be cross-matched with multiple infants. Three or more infants may be cross-matched with and receive aliquots of a single part *IF* they receive transfusions concurrently. Mixing plasma and packed cells at a 1:2 ratio will yield a hematocrit reading of about 45%. Test the hematocrit value after adding plasma.

5. All blood should be filtered.

51

Exchange Transfusion

A. SELECTION OF BLOOD FOR EXCHANGE TRANSFUSION

Use fresh blood less than 48 hours old. Blood stored in citrate-phosphate-dextrose longer than 48 to 72 hours may have an unacceptable serum potassium concentration, increased acid load, and decreased 2,3-DPG content.

1. For Rh Hemolytic Disease, Select Blood as Follows:

a. If the baby's ABO group is unknown, suspend group O, Rh-negative packed cells in AB fresh-frozen plasma.

b. If the baby's blood group is known prepare blood as shown in Table 51-1.

2. ABO Hemolytic Disease

a. Criteria for this disease are an O mother with an A, B, or AB infant, an A mother with a B infant, or a B mother with an A infant, positive direct Coombs test result in the infant.

b. Use group O, Rh-specific, packed cells cross-matched with

TABLE 51-1.—BLOOD PREPARATIONS FOR BABIES WITH KNOWN BLOOD TYPE

BLOOD TYPE		
MOTHER	BABY	GIVE BABY
A	A	A Rh negative whole blood
O	O	O Rh negative whole blood
O	A	O Rh negative cells in AB plasma
O	B	O Rh negative cells in AB plasma
AB	A	A Rh negative whole blood
AB	B	B Rh negative whole blood

both mother and infant serum specimens, accompanied by group-specific fresh-frozen plasma.

3. **Hyperbilirubinemia, Negative Direct Coombs Test Result, or Exchange Transfusion in Infant With Sepsis or Hyperammonemia** Use group-specific, RH-specific, whole blood.

B. TECHNIQUE

1. Exchange transfusion may be performed through an umbilical venous catheter, via an inferior vena cava catheter placed from a peripheral vein, or by simultaneous infusion through an umbilical venous catheter and withdrawal from an umbilical arterial catheter.

2. General Conditions

a. Evacuate gastric contents and restrain the infant under a radiant warmer. Place the infant on cardiorespiratory monitor.

b. Use asceptic technique in placing catheters and throughout the procedure.

c. Nurse should monitor and record heart rate, respiratory rate, temperature, behavior, volume of blood infused, and volume removed throughout the exchange.

3. Catheter Placement

a. Catheter should ideally be placed through the ductus venosus into the inferior vena cava with the tip at the level of the diaphragm. It should not lie in the pulmonary, hepatic, or portal veins, as pressure from infusion or injection of calcium may cause damage.

b. Location of the tip of the catheter should be verified roentgenographically before exchange transfusion; if it is technically impossible to pass the catheter through the ductus venosus, exchange transfusion should be performed with the catheter removed as far as possible and still obtaining blood return.

4. Procedure

a. Blood should be warmed to 37.5°C in blood warmer. Mix blood periodically during the procedure to prevent settling.

b. Normally, a double-volume exchange transfusion is performed (one volume = 80 ml/kg for term infants and 90–100 ml/kg for preterm infants).

c. Exchange increments (syringe size) vary from 5 ml in the smallest unstable infant to 20 ml in a term infant.

d. Initially, withdraw the first increment and save for laboratory tests (hematocrit, total/direct bilirubin, calcium, etc.). Then transfuse with an equal amount.

e. Do not leave infant with a deficit unless there is evidence of congestive heart failure (enlarged liver, high central venous pressure).

f. Calcium gluconate 10%, 0.5 to 1.0 ml, may be given slowly after every 100 to 150 ml of blood if the infant is jittery or has a low preexchange calcium level.

g. Velocity of replacement is important. A slow (one- to 2-hour) procedure is probably more efficient in removing bilirubin from tissue stores and is safer.

h. As an alternative to venous exchange, blood may be simultaneously infused into the venous catheter and removed from an umbilical artery catheter using 30- to 50-ml syringes and two operators.

i. Infusion through the umbilical artery should be avoided since spinal injuries due to microemboli may occur.

j. Postexchange specimen:
   i. Send to blood bank for cross-match with new blood donor for subsequent exchange transfusion.
   ii. Send to laboratory for hematocrit, total/direct bilirubin, binding tests, platelets, calcium, sodium, potassium, and glucose analysis.

k. *Volume deficit*—Except for severely hydropic infants, erythroblastotic infants have near-normal blood volumes, and high central venous pressures are usually the result of acid-base imbalance. However, donor blood has a high plasma protein concentration compared with that of premature or erythroblastotic infants. This may result in fluid shifts and volume overload that may not be apparent until after the procedure is over. Careful monitoring of central venous pressure, limited exchange transfusion with packed cells, and appropriate adjustment of vascular volume by leaving a volume deficit may be required in severely affected newborns.

C. EFFICIENCY

1. A two-volume exchange transfusion will remove about 90% of the circulating fetal RBCs.

2. The postexchange bilirubin concentration will usually be about one half the preexchange value and will typically rebound to about two thirds the initial concentration. If the postexchange bilirubin concentration is higher than two thirds the preexchange level, a large extravascular reservoir of bilirubin probably exists, and an additional exchange will almost always be required within hours.

D. POSTPROCEDURAL CARE

1. Observe the infant for evidence of heart failure, enlarging liver, tachycardia, arrhythmias, tachypnea, and abdominal distention.

2. If the condition is stable, feed the baby two to four hours after procedure.

3. Monitor the blood glucose level (Dextrostix) for two hours after the exchange.

4. Check the bilirubin concentration for postexchange rebound four hours after the exchange. This value should provide baseline for evaluating the subsequent rate of rise of serum bilirubin.

E. COMPLICATIONS ARE INFREQUENT, BUT INCLUDE THE FOLLOWING:

1. Cardiac arrest due to hyperkalemia, hypocalcemia, citrate toxicity, air embolization, volume overload, and arrhythmias.

2. Vascular complications due to air or clot embolization, thrombosis, phlebitis, tissue necrosis from calcium infusion, and necrotizing enterocolitis (colonic perforation).

3. Electrolyte imbalance from hyperkalemia, hypernatremia, hypocalcemia, and acidosis.

4. Hemorrhage from heparin, thrombocytopenia, and vessel perforation.

5. Infection from hepatitis, CMV, or bacteria.

6. Miscellaneous complications from mechanical injury to donor cells, transfusion reaction, graft vs. host syndrome, and reactive hypoglycemia.

52

Peritoneal Dialysis

A. INDICATIONS

1. Renal Failure in Association With the Following:

a. Severe hyperkalemia (serum potassium level greater than 7.5 mEq/L, presence of ECG abnormalities, or both)

b. Severe acidosis (serum bicarbonate level less than 12 mEq/L) and azotemia (BUN level greater than 75 mg/dl)

c. Volume overload with congestive failure, hypertension, or massive edema

2. Other

a. Hyperammonemia

b. Drug overdosage

B. SELECTION AND PREPARATION OF DIALYSIS SOLUTIONS

1. Peritoneal dialysis is performed with commercially available dialysate solutions warmed to body temperatuare prior to usage. Patients with significant lactic acidosis, which may occur in the presence of liver disease and hypoxia/hypoperfusion and which is initially identified by an elevated anion gap, should not be dialyzed with solutions containing lactate. A bicarbonate dialysis solution may be used with the necessary calcium provided parenterally.

a. Heparin, 1 unit/ml, should be added to the first 100 to 200 ml.

b. A 1.5% glucose solution should be used initially.

c. Higher glucose concentrations can be used if fluid removal has been inadequate with lower concentrations. Severe hyperglycemia may occur with high dextrose–containing dialysate solutions.

2. Normokalemic patients should have potassium (3.5 mEq/L) added to dialysate solution, while hyperkalemic patients should be initially treated without added potassium until serum values return to normal.

C. PROCEDURE

1. Catheter Placement

a. A 14-gauge intracath with three side holes added, or a pediatric dialysis trocar catheter shortened if necessary by cutting the tip to ensure that side holes remain in the peritoneum, is used.

b. If long-term dialysis is anticipated, a Tenckhoff catheter is preferred.

c. Place the catheter through surgically prepared area in the left lower or right lower quadrant.

d. Connect the catheter to an extension tube, a "Y" connector, and to a clamped tube leading to the dialysate and evacuation bottles. Maintain a closed system and change tubing and bottle every 12 hours. A commercially available peritoneal dialysis kit is usually used to supply the needed tubing and connectors.

2. Dialysate is infused by gravity, using a dwell time of 30 to 45 minutes. Fluid is then removed by gravity.

3. Small exchange volumes should be used in the range of 20 to 30 ml/kg, since large volumes can compromise ventilation.

4. The infant should be weighed two to four times daily. Strict recording of the patient's weight, intake, and output must be maintained.

5. Serum sodium, potassium, and glucose values should be monitored every two to six hours, and routine chemistry studies performed every 24 hours. Calcium should be monitored closely, if bicarbonate diagnosis is used.

6. Antibiotics may be provided in the dialysate at the first sign of peritonitis or to maintain levels in infants who are already receiving antibiotics.

D. COMPLICATIONS

1. **Infections**   Gram stain and culture solutions every 12 to 24 hours.

2. **Fluid Overload**   Increase the amount of glucose in the dialysate to 2.59 gm/dl and monitor the blood glucose level carefully. Occasionally 4.25 gm/dl glucose is required.

3. **Hyperglycemia**   may require insulin, ¼ unit every four hours or as needed to maintain normal glucose levels.

4. **Hypokalemia**   Increase the amount of potassium in the dialysate.

53

Radionuclide Evaluation of the Critically Ill Newborn

A. TECHNICAL CONSIDERATIONS

1. **Instrumentation** Imaging studies in newborn infants are performed with a permanent or portable gamma scintillation camera equipped with computers for quantitative analysis, image manipulation, or both.

2. **Radiopharmaceuticals** The absorbed dose per megacurie administered increases with decreasing body surface area, resulting in a two to four times greater radiation exposure to an infant than to an adult for the same procedure. Because of this, all requests for pediatric studies are screened to ensure that the procedure is designed to yield maximum clinical information.

B. RADIONUCLIDE EVALUATION OF PULMONARY DISEASE

1. Radiopharmaceuticals and Techniques

a. *Ventilation scan.*—If the infant is intubated, Xenon-133 gas is administered via the endotracheal tube. Otherwise, Xenon-133 in saline is given by IV injection. Abnormalities of ventilation include restrictive changes with delayed wash-in of activity and obstruction with delayed trapping of Xenon-133 in the lungs.

b. *Perfusion scan.*—Technetium-99m MAA (microaggregates of albumin) is injected intravenously. Albumin aggregates lodge in the pulmonary capillaries in a pattern of distribution that is proportional to pulmonary arterial blood flow.

c. *Interpretation.*—Combined ventilatory and perfusion images demonstrate the distribution of air and blood within the lung and provide information regarding regional pulmonary function. Abnormal studies can be classified into two categories:

   i. Unmatched perfusion defect, which implies a circulatory abnormality (rare in neonates).

   ii. Matched ventilation-perfusion defect, which indicates pulmonary parenchymal disease (most common finding in neonates).

2. **Scintigraphic Findings** may be helpful in the following instances:

   a. Pulmonary sequestration

   b. Congenital or acquired lobar emphysema

   c. Congenital hypoplastic lung

   d. Bronchopulmonary dysplasia

   e. Laryngeal, tracheal, or bronchial obstruction

C. RADIONUCLIDE EVALUATION OF GASTROINTESTINAL TRACT DISEASE

1. Liver-Spleen Scan

   a. *Technique.*—Localization of intravenously injected technetium Tc 99m sulfur colloid is dependent on phagocytosis by liver and spleen.

   b. *Uses.*—Birth trauma with suspected rupture of liver or spleen; evaluation of infants with dextrocardia and suspected asplenia or polysplenia.

2. Iodine-133 Rose Bengal

   a. *Technique.*—The radiopharmaceutical is injected intravenously and all stool specimens are collected for 72 hours. Less than 10% fecal excretion over 24 hours suggests biliary atresia. There is a 20% false-positive rate, however, in patients with neonatal hepatitis.

   b. *Use.*—Differentiation of neonatal hepatitis from biliary atresia or choledochal cysts.

3. Technetium-99m Pyrophosphate

   a. *Technique.*—The radiopharmaceutical is injected intravenously and 2½-hour delayed images of the abdomen are obtained. A positive study is defined as a curvilinear focus of increased activity anterior to the kidneys and spine. Positive studies have been observed in infants with full-thickness ischemic infarcts of the bowel.

b. *Uses.*—Assessment of infants with suspected necrotizing enterocolitis.

4. Technetium-99m Sulfur Colloid Milk Scans

a. *Technique.*—Infants are given the tracer in milk, formula, or water, and serial one-minute images are obtained for one hour. A positive study is defined as two or more visible episodes of esophageal reflux.

b. *Uses.*—Recurrent emesis and aspiration pneumonia due to suspected gastroesophageal reflux.

5. Technetium-99m Pertechnetate Scan

a. *Technique.*—Pertechnetate is secreted by the parietal cells of the gastric mucosa, including ectopic mucosa associated with Meckel's diverticula. Patients are imaged for 60 minutes following injection. Focal areas of increased uptake discrete from the stomach are abnormal.

b. *Uses.*—Meckel's diverticulum, persistence of the proximal omphalomesenteric duct.

D. RADIONUCLIDE EVALUATION OF THE URINARY TRACT

1. Radiopharmaceuticals and Techniques

a. *Technetium-99m DTPA.*—This radiopharmaceutical is cleared by glomerular filtration following IV injection. Rapid dynamic images of renal blood flow delayed static images provide information regarding renal size, shape, function, and the presence or absence of urinary obstruction.

b. *Iodohippurate sodium (I-131).*—This agent is rapidly cleared by tubular secretion, and uptake by the kidney is proportional to effective renal blood flow. Iodohippurate curve is generated over each kidney by computer manipulation of scintigraphic data. Effective renal plasma flow and tubular functions can be assessed.

2. Uses

a. Differential diagnosis of enlarged kidney(s)
  i. Hydronephrosis
  ii. Duplicated kidney
  iii. Horseshoe kidney
  iv. Multicystic kidney

v. Polycystic kidneys
vi. Wilms' tumor
vii. Adrenal tumor
viii. Downward displacement of normal-sized kidney
ix. Renal vein thrombosis

b. Other conditions
   i. *Renal agenesis.*—Scans show no functioning renal parenchyma.
   ii. Renovascular hypertension secondary to renal artery thrombosis. Iodohippurate sodium I-131 with computer analysis shows reduced effective renal plasma flow, increased water resorption, and prolonged tubular transport time in the affected kidney.

E. RADIONUCLIDE EVALUATION OF THE SKELETAL SYSTEM

1. **Technique**   Technetium-99m MDP is injected intravenously, and delayed images of the skeleton are obtained 2½ hours after injection.

2. **Uses**   The detection of osteomyelitis and its differentiation from septic arthritis and cellulitis.

3. **Limitations**   A 0% to 30% rate of false-negative bone scans occurs in infants with osteomyelitis.

4. **Gallium Citrate (GA-67)**   Because of its high radiation dose, we prefer not to use this agent in neonates.

F. RADIONUCLIDE EVALUATION OF LEFT-TO-RIGHT CARDIAC SHUNTS

1. **Technique**   Technetium-99m DTPA is rapidly injected into the superficial jugular vein, and dynamic images of the heart and lungs are acquired. A curve is generated over the lung which measures radioactivity as it appears in and leaves the pulmonary circulation. Using a curve-fitting program, a ratio of pulmonary to systemic-flow is generated. Ratios greater than 1.2:1 indicate left-to-right shunting.

2. **Uses**   Examination of infants with patent ductus arteriosus and other forms of congenital heart disease.

G. BLOOD VOLUME DETERMINATIONS

1. **Technique**   The RBCs from 2 ml of the infant's blood are labeled with sodium pertechnetate (Tc-99m). One milliliter of labeled RBCs is reinjected into the patient, and a 2-ml blood sample is drawn from another vein 20 minutes later. Red cell mass is then calculated based on the dilution of tracer in the infant's circulation.

2. **Uses**   Blood loss, polycythemia.

54

Infant Transport

A. REGIONALIZATION OF NEONATAL CARE

1. Rural (primary) and community (secondary) facilities may need to transfer sick infants to regional (tertiary) centers for special care. (Maternal transport is generally preferred but not always feasible.) Ground transportation is used for most transports within 100 miles. Air transport is more efficient for longer distances.

2. Following initial resuscitation of a sick infant, referring physicians are encouraged to contact their tertiary center and the attending neonatologist, or other specialists, for consultation or patient referral. A 24-hour "hotline" is often available for this service.

B. STABILIZATION FOR TRANSPORT

Steps taken by the transport team to stabilize infants for and during transport may differ from those normally taken in the care of an inborn infant, but the goals are similar.

1. **Initial History and Physical Examination** should provide the major diagnosis or diagnoses.

2. **Circulation** Pretransport assessment should include BP determination, assessment of capillary filling, blood volume, and a hematocrit reading. Therapy for hypoperfusion should be initiated before transport.

3. **Oxygenation and Ventilation**

   a. The goal is to maintain the arterial oxygen tension between 50 and 80 torr and the arterial carbon dioxide tensions between 35 and 45 torr during transport.

   b. If available, transcutaneous oxygen and carbon dioxide monitors should be used.

   c. Team members may have to rely on their clinical assessment and provide enough oxygen to relieve central cyanosis.

   d. Criteria for ventilatory assistance during transport are more lenient than in the neonatal intensive care unit in order to ensure a safer transport and should be individualized in consultation with the responsible neonatologist.

4. Glucose Homeostasis

   a. Parenteral glucose infusion at 4 to 6 mg/kg/min or greater is indicated if the patient is normoglycemic, and at 8 mg/kg/min if the patient has been hypoglycemic.

   b. During transport, Dextrostix monitoring should be continued and the glucose infusion rate adjusted to maintain an estimated glucose concentration of 40 to 120 mg/dl.

5. Sepsis/Meningitis
If infection is suspected, evaluation and initiation of treatment should normally be begun before transporting the infant.

6. Thermal protection

   a. Prewarm the transport module and pad.

   b. You may also place an inner heat shield in the transport module or wrap the infant in thin plastic blankets.

   c. Minimize the time outside the warmer or incubator. Manipulate the infant through the portals only.

   d. If the infant is already hypothermic, rewarming is accomplished by setting the module air temperature a maximum of 1.5°C above the abdominal skin temperature. Gooseneck lamps should not be used. Warm water bottles (surgical gloves filled with warm water) may be used cautiously providing direct skin contact is avoided.

   e. If the infant is hypothermic, measure an initial rectal temperature and follow as necessary.

7. Gastrointestinal Decompression
Infants with vomiting or abdominal distention or who are at risk for aspiration should have a nasogastric tube placed for decompression prior to transport.

8. For Specific Stabilization Procedures
see appropriate sections.

9. Talk to the Parents
and show them the infant before leaving the referring hospital.

55

Neonatal Drug Formulary

DRUG	ROUTE	DOSAGE	COMMENTS
Albumin 25%	IV	1.0 gm/kg (4 ml/kg)	Repeat as necessary monitoring BP. Usually diluted 1:4 with saline before use
Alphamethyldopa (Aldomet)	IV	20–40 mg/kg/day divided q 6–8 hr	IV for hypertensive crisis only. Dilute 1–20 mg/ml and infuse over 30–60 min
	Orally	Initial: 10 mg/kg/day divided q 6–12 hr. Maximum 40 mg/kg/day	
Aminophylline	IV	5 mg/kg loading dose, 7–12 mg/kg/day divided q 6–12 hr	Monitor serum levels to maintain 6–13 µg/ml
Amphotericin B	IV	0.25 mg/kg/day. In single dose over 6 hr (Dilute in 5% D/W, concentration not to exceed 10 mg/dl). Increase daily as tolerated to 1 mg/kg/day	See manufacturer's package insert. Renal and hematologic toxicity
Ampicillin	IV	Initial dosage: < 1 wk, 100 mg/kg/day divided q 12 hr; > 1 week, 200 mg/kg/day divided q 8 hr. Continuing dosage: documented sepsis. < 1 week, 50 mg/kg/day q 12 hr; > 1 week, 100 mg/kg/day every 8 hr	

Atropine	SC/IV/IM	0.01–0.03 mg/kg/dose	
Bethanechol	Orally	0.6 mg/kg/day divided q 6–8 hr	
Caffeine citrate	Orally	20 mg/kg/loading dose, 10 mg/kg/day divided q 12 hr	Monitor blood levels to maintain 8–15 µg/ml
Calcium gluceptate	IV	110–220 mg/kg dose	Infuse over 5–10 min
Calcium gluconate (10%)	IV	0.5–1.0 ml/kg	Infuse slowly over 5–10 min. Monitor heart rate
Cefotaxime	IV/IM	100–200 mg/kg/dose (1–2 ml/kg) Documented meningitis: continue initial dosage.	
		<1 week, 50 mg/kg/dose q 12 hr.	
		>1 week, 50 mg/kg/dose q 8 hr.	
Chloramphenicol	Orally or IV	<1 week, 25 mg/kg/day; >1 week, 50 mg/kg/day divided q 12 hr	Monitor blood levels
Cortisone acetate	IM/orally	Physiological replacement, 0.7 mg/kg/day po divided q 8 hr; pharmacologic dose, 2.5–10 mg/kg/day divided q 8 hr	
(Defibrillation)	"Paddles"	2.5 watt-sec/kg	
Desoxycortisone acetate (DOCA)	IM	1–5 mg q 24 hr	Adjust according to electrolyte level

Continued.

DRUG	ROUTE	DOSAGE	COMMENTS
Dexamethasone	IM/IV/orally	0.1–1.0 mg/kg/dose q 6–8 hr	Higher dose for short-term trial in brain edema or chronic lung disease
Diazepam (Valium)	IM/IV/orally	0.1–0.4 mg/kg/dose	Titrate carefully to control seizures. Risk for circulatory and respiratory depression.
Digoxin	Orally	TDD Premature infant: 35 μg/kg over 12–24 hr, divided doses, ½ stat, ¼ 6–12 hr, ¼ 6–12 hr later. Term: 50–70 μg/kg give total dose over 12–48 hr, divided doses, ½, ¼, ¼. Maintenance dose: ¼ to ⅓ of TDD per day q 12 hr	TDD = total digitalizing dose
	IV	⅔ of oral dose	

Drug	Route	Dose	Comments
Dopamine HCl	IV infusion	2–5 µg/kg/min. Increase up to 15 µg/kg/min as indicated	Titrate BP. Dilute 1 ml of 40 mg/ml dopamine in 250 ml of 5% dextrose or normal saline solution giving a concentration of 160 µg/ml. Infusion rate of 1 ml/kg/hr will deliver 2.7 µg/kg/min
Dobutamine	IV infusion	Same as dopamine	Limited experience in newborns
Edrophonium chloride (Tensilon)	IV	Give 0.05 mg/kg initially. Repeat at 1-minute intervals to total dose of 0.2 mg/kg	If adverse reaction, give atropine, 0.01–0.04 mg/kg/dose
Epinephrine	IV	0.1 ml/kg/dose using aqueous 1:10,000 solution (0.1 mg/ml).	
	IV infusion	0.5–1.5 µg/kg/min	
Furosemide (Lasix)	IM/IV	1–2 mg/kg/dose every 4–12 hr	Refractory CHF or hypotension: 4 ampules of 1:1000 in 250 ml DSW. Run at 2–6 ml/kg/hr
	Orally	2–5 mg/kg/dose every 6–12 hrs	
Gentamicin sulfate	IV	3.0 mg/kg q 24 hr if <2,000 gm and <1 wk of age; 2.5 mg/kg q 12 hr for all other neonates 2.5 mg/kg q 8 hr for infants >28 days of age	Monitor serum potassium, chloride Absorption variable Monitor levels and adjust dosage accordingly
Glucagon	IM	300 µg/kg/dose up to a total dose of 1 mg	

Continued.

DRUG	ROUTE	DOSAGE	COMMENTS
Heparin sodium	IV infusion	0.5–1.0 units per ml of IV fluid	Add to all IV solutions infused through arterial lines
Hydralazine HCl	Orally IV	0.3–3 mg/kg/day divided q 6 hr 0.15 mg/kg every 10 min until drop in BP or maximum dose 1–4 mg/kg/day.	Hypertensive care
Hydrocortisone (Solucortef)	IV/IM/orally	Pharmacologic: 10 mg/kg/day divided q 6 hr. Maintenance: 1 mg/kg/day	
Insulin	SC/IV	Glycosuria with IV alimentation ¼ unit/kg q 4–6 hr prn or 0.1–0.2 units/kg/hr continuous infusion	
Isoproterenol (Isuprel)	IV infusion	0.2–0.5 µg/kg/min	Ampules contain 1 mg/5 cc (1:5000). 2 mg in 200 ml D5/W at rate of 1.0 ml/kg/hr delivers 0.17 µg/kg/min. Titrate according to BP
Kanamycin sulfate	IM	<1 wk, 10–20 mg/kg/day divided every 12 hr; >1 wk, 20–30 mg/kg/day divided q 8–12 hr	Lower dosage for smaller infants
Kayexalate	Orally/PR	1 gm/kg (25% solution = 4 cc/kg) every 6 hr	

Magnesium sulfate	IV/IM	25–50 mg/kg/dose × 3–4 doses prn	Provided as 50 gm/dl solution (1 gm/2 ml)
Mannitol	IV infusion	1.0–1.5 gm/kg/dose (5–7.5 ml/kg/dose). Repeat q 8–12 hr prn	Given as 20 gm/dl solution over 20–30 min
Metaclopramide	Orally	0.1 mg/kg/dose, 1–4 times/day	
Morphine sulfate	SC/IV	0.05–0.1 mg/kg/dose prn	
Mycostatin (nystatin)	Orally	100,000 units q 6 hr	
Nafcillin	IV/IM	<1 wk, 100 mg/kg/day divided q 12 hr. >1 wk, 200 mg/kg/day divided q 6 hr	
Naloxone (Narcan)	IM/IV	0.01 mg/kg/dose, repeat as necessary	
Neomycin	Orally	90 mg/kg/day divided q 6 hr	
Neostigmine (Prostigmine)	IM/SC	0.04 mg/kg/dose	Antidote: Atropine, 0.01–0.04 mg/kg/dose
Pancuronium (Pavulon)	IV	Initial dose, 0.05 mg/kg Subsequent: 0.01–0.05 mg/kg q 2–6 hr prn	Antidote: Neostigmine, 0.04–0.07 mg/kg, and atropine 0.02 mg/kg (no sooner than 30 min after pancuronium)
Penicillin G	IV/IM	<1 wk, 50,000 units/kg/day q 12 hr. >1 wk, 75,000 units/kg/day q 8 hr	

Continued.

287

DRUG	ROUTE	DOSAGE	COMMENTS
Pentobarbital (Nembutal)	IM	3 mg/kg/dose	Sedation for procedures
Phenobarbital	IV/IM	Loading dose: 10–20 mg/kg IV or IM.	Monitor serum level to maintain 20–30 µg/ml
	IV/IM/PO	Maintenance: 5 mg/kg/day divided every 12 hr	
Phenytoin (Dilantin)	IV	Loading dose: 15–20 mg/kg/IV	Give in increments of 5 mg/kg every 15–20 min; maximum rate IV = 0.5 mg/kg/min. Compatible with normal saline only
		Maintenance: 5–8 mg/kg/day divided q 12 hr	Oral doses poorly absorbed
Pitressin aqueous	SC	0.125–0.5 ml/dose q 6–8 hr	Aqueous = 20 units/ml
oil	IM	0.2 ml/dose q 1–3 days	Oil = 5 units/ml (shake well) Titrate effect
Prednisone	Orally	Pharmacologic, 1–5 mg/kg/day divided q 6 hr	⅕ of cortisone dose. Higher dose for short-term trial in chronic lung disease
Procainamide	IV	1.5–2.0 mg/kg in IV drip over 20–30 min	For ventricular arrhythmia; titrate and repeat as necessary
Propranolol HCl	Orally	0.5–1.0 mg/kg/day divided q 6 hr.	For ventricular tachycardia, supraventricular arrhythmias.

	Route	Dose	Comments
	IV	0.01–0.2 mg/kg single dose over 10 min. May repeat in 10 min	Toxic reaction: hypotension bronchospasm
Protamine sulfate	IV	0.5–1.0 mg per 100 units of heparin given during previous 3 hr	Do not exceed 50 mg
Pyridostigmine	Orally	5 mg/kg/24 hr (30 min before feeding divided q 6 hr)	
	IM	0.05–0.15 mg/dose (30 min before feeding) q 6 hr	
Pyridoxine	IM/IV	50 mg/dose	For intractable seizures
Quinidine	IV	2–10 mg/kg/dose. Repeat q 3–6 hr prn	For refractory supraventricular tachycardia secondary to digoxin
Sodium bicarbonate	IV/Orally	2–3 mEq/kg/dose over 5–10 min	Commonly provided as 44 mEq/50 ml. Dilute 1:1 or 1:2 with water or DW "½ correction" (mEq) = Base deficit × 0.3 × body wt (kg)
Spironolactone (Aldactone)	Orally	1–3 mg/kg/day divided q 6–12 hr	
Theophylline	Orally	Loading dose: 4 mg/kg; maintenance dose: 6–10 mg/kg/day divided q 6–12 hr;	
L-Thyroxine	IV/IM/Orally	20 μg/day	Monitor serum levels to maintain 6–13 μ/ml. Toxic effects: tachycardia, vomiting Monitor T_4

Continued.

DRUG	ROUTE	DOSAGE	COMMENTS
Tolazoline HCl (Priscoline)	IV	1 mg/kg, bolus—if no response, repeat in 10 min. If response, continue with infusion 1–2 mg/kg/hr	Scalp vein preferable. Generally see tolazoline flush. Monitor BP.
Tromethamine (THAM)	IV	Packaged as 0.3 mEq/ml solution. Same dose as sodium bicarbonate	May cause hyperkalemia or hypoglycemia. Contraindicated in renal failure

56

Glossary of Abbreviations

ABG	Arterial blood gas
AGA	Appropriate for gestational age
Alk-Phos	Alkaline phosphatase
Ao	Aortic
ATN	Acute tubular necrosis
AUBC	Apparent unbound bilirubin concentration
AV	Atrioventricular
BAEP	Brain-stem auditory evoked potential
BCAA	Branched-chain amino acid
BP	Blood pressure
BPD	Biparietal diameter
	Bronchopulmonary dysplasia
BUN	Blood urea nitrogen
BW	Body weight
CBG	Capillary blood gas
CHF	Congestive heart failure
CIE	Counterimmunoelectrophoresis
CLD	Chronic lung disease
CMV	Cytomegalovirus
CNP	Continuous negative pressure
CNS	Central nervous system
CPAP	Continuous positive airway pressure
CPIP	Chronic pulmonary insufficiency of prematurity
CSF	Cerebrospinal fluid
CST	Contraction stress test
CT	Computed axial tomography
CVH	Combined ventricular hypertrophy
CVP	Central venous pressure
D/C	Discontinue
DES	Diethylstilbesterol
DIC	Disseminated intravascular clotting
DOCA	Deoxycorticosterone acetate
DRIP	Diuretic responsive interstitial pneumopathy
DTR	Deep tendon reflexes
E_3	Estriol
ECMO	Extracorporeal membranes oxygenators

ECW	Extracellular water
EEG	Electroencephalogram
ELISA	Enzyme-linked immunosorbant assay
EM	Electron microscopy
ET	Endotracheal
	Ejection time
Et	Expiratory time
FHR	Fetal heart rate
FSI	Foam stability index
GASA	Growth-adjusted sonographic age
GFR	Glomerular filtration rate
GGT	Gamma glutamyl transferase
GI	Gastrointestinal
HCM	Health care maintenance
HCS	Human chorionic somatomammotrophin
Hct	Hematocrit
HDN	Hemolytic disease of the newborn
Hgb	Hemoglobin
HMD	Hyaline membrane disease
HPF	High power field
HPL	Human placental lactogen
H-T	Head to trunk ratio
ICW	Intracellular water
i.d.	Inner diameter
IDM	Infant of diabetic mother
I/E	Inspiratory to expiratory ratio
IM	Intramuscular
It	Inspiratory time
IUGR	Intrauterine growth retardation
IVH	Intraventricular hemorrhage
IVS	Intraventricular septal thickness
KUB	Kidneys, ureter, and bladder
LA	Left atrium
LAD	Left atrial diameter
LGA	Large for gestational age
L/S	Lecithin to sphingomyelin ratio
LV	Left ventricle
LVED	Left ventricular end diastolic
LVES	Left ventricular end systolic
LVH	Left ventricular hypertrophy
LVPW	Left ventricular posterior wall
MPA	Main pulmonary artery
NEC	Necrotizing enterocolitis
NG	Nasogastric
NS	Normal saline
NST	Non-stress testing
OCT	Oxtocin challenge test
o.d.	Outer diameter

OD	Optical density
OFC	Occipital-frontal circumference
PAC	Premature atrial contraction
PAPP-A	Pregnancy-associated plasma protein A
PAT	Paroxysmal atrial tachycardia
PDA	Patent ductus arteriosus
PEEP	Positive end-expiratory pressure
PEP	Pre-ejection period
	Phosphoenol pyruvate
PFC	Persistence of fetal circulation
PG	Phosphatidyl glycerol
PIE	Pulmonary interstitial emphysema
PMN	Polymorphonuclear
PP5	Placental protein 5
PROM	Premature rupture of the membranes
PT	Prothrombin time
PTC	Persistent transitional circulation
PTT	Partial thromboplastin time
PVC	Premature ventricular contraction
PVS	Percussion, vibration, and suctioning
RA	Right atrium
RAH	Right atrial hypertrophy
RBC	Red blood cell
RDS	Respiratory distress syndrome
RLF	Retrolental fibroplasia
RV	Right ventricle
RVH	Right ventricular hypertrophy
SD	Standard deviation
SGA	Small for gestational age
SGOT	Serum glutamic oxaloacetate transaminase
SGPT	Serum glutamic pyruvic transaminase
STI	Systolic T intervals
SVT	Supraventricular tachycardia
TB	Tuberculosis
TBG	Thyroid-binding globulin
TEF	Tracheoesophageal fistula
THAM	Tris-hydroxymethyl aminomethane
TIUV	Total intrauterine volume
TORCH	Toxoplasmosis, other, rubella, cytomegalovirus, and herpes
TPN	Total parenteral nutrition
TSH	Thyroid-stimulating hormone
UAC	Umbilical artery catheter
UGI	Upper gastrointestinal
UVC	Umbilical venous catheter
VP	Venous pressure
VSD	Ventricular septal defect
WBC	White blood cell

57

Appendix

TABLE 57–1.—HEMATOLOGY: MEAN RED CELL VALUES DURING GESTATION*

AGE (weeks)	HB (gm/dl)	HEMATOCRIT (%)	RBC (10^6/mm³)	MEAN CORPUSCLE vol (μ³)	MEAN CORPUSCLE Hb(vv)	MEAN CORPUSCLE HB conc (%)	NUC RBC (% of RBCs)	RETIC (%)
12	8.0–10.0	33	1.5	180	60	34	5.0–8.0	40
16	10.0	35	2.0	140	45	33	2.0–4.0	10–25
20	11.0	37	2.5	135	44	33	1.0	10–20
24	14.0	40	3.5	123	38	31	1.0	5–10
28	14.5	45	4.0	120	40	31	0.5	5–10
34	15.0	47	4.4	118	38	32	0.2	3–10

*From Oski F.A., Naiman J.L.: Hematologic Problems in the Newborn, ed. 2, Philadelphia, W.B. Saunders Co., 1972.

TABLE 57–2.—Approximate Neutral Thermal Environment Temperatures Weight (gms)*

AGE	<1200	1201–1500	1501–2500	>2600 (>36 weeks)
0–12 Hr	35.0	34.0	33.3	32.8
12–24 Hr	34.5	33.8	32.8	32.4
24–96 Hr	34.5	33.5	32.3	32.0
4–14 Days		33.5	32.1	31.0
2–3 Wk		33.1	31.7	30.0
3–4 Wk		32.6	31.4	
4–5 Wk		32.0	30.9	
5–6 Wk		31.4	30.4	

*From Scopes J.W., Ahmed I.: *Arch. Dis. Child.* 41:417, 1966.)

TABLE 57–3.—Serum Enzymes in Newborns

ENZYMES	AGE	IU/L
Acid phosphatase*	Birth–1 month	7.4–19.4
Alanine amino transaminase (SGPT)**	Birth–10 days	1.3–11
	Birth–1 month	0–54
Aldolase†	Birth–1 month	4–24
Alkaline phosphatase**	Birth–1 month	20–225
	1 month–3 months	73–226
Aspartate amino transaminase (SGOT)**	Birth–10 days	6–25
	Birth–1 month	0–67
Creatinine phosphokinase (CPK)	Premature	0–210
	Birth–3 weeks	22–267
	3 weeks–3 months	15–134
Gamma glutamyl transpeptidase (GGPT)‡‡	Premature	56–233
	Birth–3 weeks	0–103
	3 weeks–3 months	4–111
Lactate dehydrogenase (LDH)†	Birth–10 days	150–590
	1 day–1 month	185–404
	1 month–2 years	110–244
Leucine aminopeptidase (LAP)*	Birth–1 month	29–59
	>1 month	15–50

*From O'Brien D., Rodgerson D.O.: Interpretation of biochemical values, in Kempe C.H., Silver H.K., O'Brien D. (eds.): *Current Pediatric Diagnosis and Treatment* ed. 3., Los Altos, Ca., Lange Medical Publications.

†From Meites S. (ed.): *Pediatric Clinical Chemistry: A Survey of Normals, Methods, and Instruments,* Washington, D.C., American Association for Clinical Chemistry, 1977.

**From Sitzmann F.C.: *Arch. Kindeheilk.* (Suppl.) 57:1, 1968.

‡‡From King J., Morris M.B.: *Arch. Dis. Child.* 36:604, 1961.

TABLE 57–4.—The White Blood Cell Count and the Differential Count During the First Two Weeks of Life*

| AGE | LEUKOCYTES | NEUTROPHILES | | | EOSINOPHILS | BASOPHILS | LYMPHOCYTES | MONOCYTES |
		TOTAL	SEG	BAND				
BIRTH								
Mean	18,100	11,000	9400	1600	400	100	5500	1050
Range	9.0–30.0	6.0–26.0			20–850	0–640	2.0–11.0	0.4–3.1
Mean %	—	61	52	9	2.2	0.6	31	5.8
7 DAYS								
Mean	12,200	5,500	4700	830	500	50	5000	1100
Range	5.0–21.0	1.5–10.0			70–1100	0–250	2.0–17.0	0.3–2.7
Mean %	—	45	39	6	4.1	0.4	41	9.1
14 DAYS								
Mean	11,400	4,500	3900	630	350	50	5500	1000
Range	5.0–20.0	1.0–9.5			70–1000	0–230	2.0–17.0	0.2–2–4
Mean %	40		34	5.5	3.1	0.4	48	8.8

*From Oski F., Naiman J.: Hematologic Problems in the Newborn, Philadelphia, W.B. Saunders Co., 1966.

TABLE 57–5.—WHITE CELLS AND DIFFERENTIAL COUNTS IN PREMATURE INFANTS DURING FIRST FOUR WEEKS OF POSTPARTUM LIFE*

BIRTH WEIGHT	<1500 GM			1500–2500 GM		
Age in Weeks	1	2	4	1	2	4
Total Count (× 1000/cmm)						
Mean	16.8	15.4	12.1	13.0	10.0	8.4
Range	6.1–32.8	10.4–21.3	8.7–17.2	6.7–14.7	7.0–14.1	5.8–12.4
Percent of Total						
Polymorphs						
PMN/BANDS	.11	.11	.11	.13	.16	.13
Segmented	54	45	40	55	43	41
Unsegmented	7	6	5	8	8	6
Eosinophils	2	3	3	2	3	3
Basophils	1	1	1	1	1	1
Monocytes	6	10	10	5	9	11
Lymphocytes	30	35	41	9	36	38

*From Klaus M.H., Fanaroff A.A.: Care of the High Risk Neonate, Philadelphia, W.B. Saunders Co., 1979.

TABLE 57–6.—Coagulation Factor Levels, Screening Studies, and Fibrinolysis Times in Relation to Gestational Maturity*

FACTORS	I	II	V	VII	X	VIII	IX	XI	XIII	PLATELETS	PTT	PT	TT	FT
	mg/100 mg	Percent of Normal					Mean		Titer	×1000/cmm (+SD)	Seconds			
<1500 gm 28–32 weeks	215	21	64	42		50	—	—	—	300 (70)	117	21	—	326
1500–2000 gm 32–36 weeks	220	25	67	37		44	—	—	1/8	260 (60)	113	18	14	214
2000–2500 gm 36–40 weeks	240	35	66	48		67	—	—	1/8	325 (75)	77	17	10	214
>2500 gm Term	210	60	92	56		67	26	42	1/8	325 (70)	71	16	9	95
Mothers of premature infants	520	92	110	178		—	—	—	—	225 (45)	73	14	7	—
Mothers of term infants	500	92	110	206		196	130	69	1/16	215 (41)	75	14	8	278

PTT = Partial thromboplastin time; TT = thrombin time; PT = prothrombin time; FT = fibrinolysis time.
*From Klaus M.H, Fanaroff A.A.: Care of the High Risk Neonate. Philadelphia, W.B. Saunders Co., 1979.

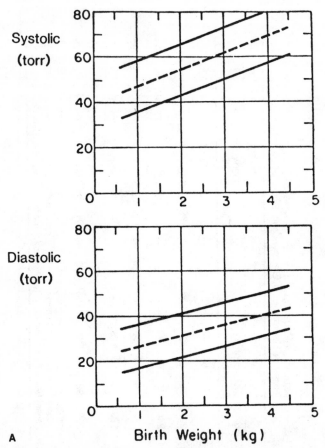

A   Birth Weight (kg)

Fig 57–1A.—Blood pressure in the first 12 hours of life. Linear regressions (broken lines) and 95% confidence limits (solid lines) of systolic (top) and diastolic (bottom) aortic blood pressures on birth weight in 61 healthy newborn infants during the first 12 hours after birth. For systolic pressure, $y = 7.13x + 40.45$; $r = .79$. For diastolic pressure, $y = 4.81x + 22.18$; $r = .71$. For both, $n = 413$ and $P < .001$. (From Versmold, et al.: Aortic blood pressure during the first 12 hours of life in infants with birth weight 610 to 4220 grams. Pediatrics 67:607, 1981. Reproduced by permission.)

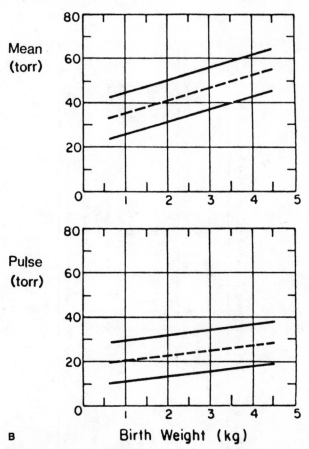

Fig 57–1B.—Blood pressure in the first 12 hours of Life. Linear regressions (broken lines) and 95% confidence limits (solid lines) of mean pressure (top) and pulse pressure (systolic-diastolic pressure amplitude) (bottom) on birth weight in 61 healthy newborn infants during the first 12 hours after birth. (From Versmold et al., Pediatrics 67:607, 1981. Reproduced by permission.)

TABLE 57-7.—CEREBROSPINAL FLUID IN HEALTHY TERM NEWBORNS

COLOR	0–24 Hours Clear or xanthochromic	1 Day Clear or xanthochromic	7 Day Clear or xanthochromic
Red blood cells/mm³	9 (0–1,070)	23 (6–630)	3 (0–48)
Polymorphonuclear leukocytes/mm³	3 (0–70)	7 (0–26)	2 (0–5)
Lymphocytes/mm³	2 (0–20)	5 (0–16)	1 (0–4)
Proteins (mg/dl)	63 (32–240)	73 (40–148)	47 (27–65)
Glucose (mg/dl)	51 (32–78)	48 (38–64)	55 (48–6)
Lactate dehydrogenase		22–73 (Birth–7 days)	

*Data from Naidoo B.T.: *S. Afr. Med. J.* 42:932, 1968; Neches W., Platt M.: *Pediatrics* 41:1097, 1968.

Index